Psychosis - From Cell to Society

Edited by Ana Starcevic

Published in London, United Kingdom

Psychosis - From Cell to Society
http://dx.doi.org/10.5772/intechopen.1005999
Edited by Ana Starcevic

Contributors
Armita Adily, Barbara C. Walsh, Cristina López-Cabezón, Elif Küçük, Esther Badugu Patrick, Feride Uysal, Jared P. Walsh, Maria Victoria Puig, Mihaela Fadgyas Stanculete, Mustafa Akkuş, Ndumiso Ginindza, Octavia Capatina, Olubunmi Fashoto, Sara Hidalgo-Nieves, Savvina Chrysostomou, Shreshth Khanna, Sibusiso Dlamini, Sotiria Moza, Stephen Allnutt, Stephen Fashoto, Sunday Oritsetimenyin Otimenyin, Thomas Gener, Tony Butler

First published in London, United Kingdom, 2025 by IntechOpen
IntechOpen is the global imprint of INTECHOPEN LIMITED, registered in England and Wales, registration number: 11086078, 167-169 Great Portland Street, London, W1W 5PF, United Kingdom

For EU product safety concerns: IN TECH d.o.o., Prolaz Marije Krucifikse Kozulić 3, 51000 Rijeka, Croatia, info@intechopen.com or visit our website at intechopen.com.

British Library Cataloguing-in-Publication Data
A catalogue record for this book is available from the British Library

Psychosis - From Cell to Society
Edited by Ana Starcevic
p. cm.
Print ISBN 978-1-83634-413-1
Online ISBN 978-1-83634-412-4
eBook (PDF) ISBN 978-1-83634-414-8

If disposing of this product, please recycle the paper responsibly.

Meet the editor

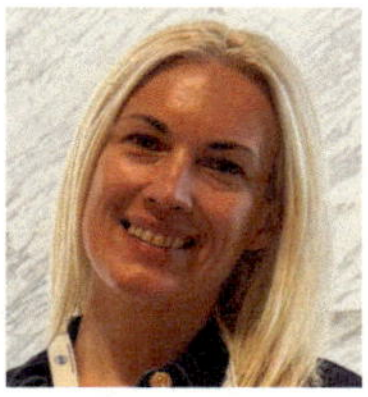

Prof. Dr. Ana Starcevic is a psychiatrist and Head of the Laboratory of Multimodal Neuroimaging at the University of Belgrade, Medical Faculty, Institute of Anatomy. Her research centers on brain morphology and functional neuroimaging, with a focus on psychiatric disorders such as depression, anxiety, and psychosis. She integrates clinical psychiatry, particularly in stress-related disorders, with advanced neuroimaging and artificial intelligence techniques. Dr. Starcevic's interdisciplinary work bridges the fields of medicine and engineering, aiming to establish a translational neuroscience approach. Her extensive publication record and use of cutting-edge imaging technologies underscore her contributions to understanding neural mechanisms underlying mental illness. A strong advocate for AI in psychiatry, she seeks to enhance diagnostic accuracy and treatment outcomes, shaping the future of personalized mental health care.

Contents

Preface

Psychosis remains a profound and multifaceted challenge, impacting not only the mental health and daily functioning of individuals but also their communities and societies at large. This book, *Psychosis – From Cell to Society*, offers a comprehensive exploration of psychosis, tracing its dimensions from neurobiological mechanisms to societal consequences, from cutting-edge diagnostic tools to the persistent challenges of early detection and stigma reduction.

The opening chapter, "The Impact of Psychosis on Mental Health and Quality of Life of an Individual", sets the stage by examining the disruptive nature of psychotic symptoms such as delusions and hallucinations and their cascading effects on emotional well-being, interpersonal relationships and societal participation. These disruptions translate into both personal suffering and economic costs, emphasizing the urgency for early and effective intervention.

Cognition lies at the heart of functionality. In "The Fog of Schizophrenia: Cognitive Impairments and Their Impact on Daily Life", the authors delve into the cognitive deficits intrinsic to schizophrenia, attention, memory, and executive dysfunction that persist despite pharmacological treatments. This chapter highlights the pressing need for cognitive remediation strategies to restore independence and improve long-term outcomes.

Understanding the biological basis of psychosis is essential for designing targeted therapies. The chapter on "Neural Substrates of Psychosis and Cognitive Impairment in Mouse Models of Schizophrenia" offers critical insights from preclinical research. Using rodent models, it investigates the neurocircuitry disrupted by psychotic processes and how pharmacological interventions variably affect prefrontal-hippocampal connectivity, offering translational relevance to human treatment.

Psychosis is not only a neuropsychiatric issue but also a cognitive-emotional phenomenon. In the perspective chapter, "Perspective Chapter: The Neuropsychological Dimension of Psychosis – Implications for Assessment and Treatment", readers are guided through the neurocognitive evaluations essential for understanding and managing psychotic disorders. It underscores the importance of modern neuropsychological tools, cognitive remediation, and culturally sensitive, evidence-based interventions.

Recognition and early intervention are cornerstones of effective mental health care. The chapter "The Role of Primary Care in Identifying Early Psychosis" stresses the vital role of frontline healthcare providers. By highlighting early warning signs and integrating primary care with specialized psychiatric services, it proposes a community-centered model for improved outcomes.

The misuse of psychoactive substances adds complexity to the clinical landscape. In "Psychoactive Substance-Induced Psychotic Disorder", the authors provide a nuanced analysis of psychosis arising from substance use. With a focus on neurobiological mechanisms, clinical features, and treatment strategies, the chapter distinguishes this form of psychosis from primary psychotic disorders, guiding clinicians in accurate diagnosis and dual-diagnosis management.

Mood instability often coexists with psychosis, as addressed in "Treatment of Hypomania". This chapter explores diagnostic challenges and outlines both pharmacologic and psychotherapeutic modalities, offering a comprehensive framework for managing this underrecognized condition within the broader spectrum of affective and psychotic disorders.

Modern challenges call for modern tools. The chapter "Mental Health Prediction Model in Eswatini Using Machine Learning Techniques" reflects a forward-looking approach by integrating artificial intelligence to predict anxiety and depression. Using national health data, it demonstrates how early identification through machine learning can pave the way for preemptive care, particularly in low-resource settings.

The impact of psychosis often extends into the criminal justice system. In "Exploring Risk Factors for Offending Behaviours in Individuals with Psychosis and Impact of Interventions to Reduce Offending", the authors explore the intersection of mental illness and criminality. Drawing from population-based research in Australia, this chapter identifies risk factors for reoffending and emphasizes the role of court diversion programs and mental health services in reducing recidivism.

Beyond neurobiology and diagnosis lies the social reality of stigma. "Perspective Chapter: The Interplay of Stigma and Psychosis", takes a critical look at how societal misconceptions intensify suffering, impede help-seeking, and limit recovery. It proposes educational, technological, and psychosocial strategies to mitigate stigma and empower individuals with psychosis.

Together, these chapters provide an integrative and holistic view of psychosis—from cells to society, from symptoms to systems of care. This book is designed not only for clinicians and researchers but also for students, policymakers, and advocates who seek to understand and transform the way we perceive and treat psychotic disorders. In a world increasingly shaped by data, technology, and social complexity, a multifaceted approach to psychosis is more essential than ever.

Let this work serve as a call to action—toward earlier detection, better treatment, reduced stigma, and ultimately, fuller lives for those affected by psychosis.

Ana Starcevic, MD, PhD
Psychiatrist,
Medical Faculty,
Institute of Anatomy,
University of Belgrade,
Belgrade, Serbia

Section 1

The Human Face of Psychosis

Chapter 1

The Impact of Psychosis on Mental Health and Quality of Life of an Individual

Shreshth Khanna

Abstract

Psychosis is a severe and a complicated mental disorder that affects the overall well-being of an individual through alterations in thought and perceptions wherein the person losses touch with reality. The symptomatology of the disorder is demarcated as positive and the negative symptoms. The positive symptoms including delusions, illusions, auditory hallucinations, and thought disorders are the additional behaviors that develop after an individual develops the illness whereas the negative symptoms include introverted behavior, poor sociability, emotional blunting, amotivation, and cognitive deficits that reflect a decline in the normal functioning capacity of the person. People with psychotic disorders exhibit a significant reduction in the overall quality of life particularly in the domains of physical and mental health, social intercourses, self-esteem, and interpersonal relationships. Psychotic disorders are also one of the leading causes of disability and disability adjusted life years (DALYs) globally, causing a dent in the economy of a country through the inherent direct healthcare costs and the indirect costs (productivity and income losses) causing a depletion in capital and labor resource pool and subsequently causing a decrease in the overall productive capacity of the country. The existing literature highlights the importance of early interventions in psychosis, community-based multidisciplinary approaches including cognitive behavior therapy, somatic interventions, and pharmacotherapy in curtailing the impact and ameliorating the overall quality of life in people with psychosis.

Keywords: psychosis, quality of life, mental health, community based services, social isolation, economic losses, psychotic disorders

1. Introduction

Psychosis is a complex mental health condition characterized by disruptions in thought processes, perception, and emotional regulation. Psychosis is a mental health condition characterized by a disconnection from reality. It can manifest in various forms. Understanding the symptoms of psychosis is vital for diagnosis, treatment, and appropriate management of the disorder. Psychosis may be a sequel to various pre-existing psychiatric, neuropsychiatric, neurologic, and neurodevelopmental conditions. Psychosis, often associated with severe mental health conditions, can lead to significant societal stigma that affects individuals, their families, and communities. This stigma can have detrimental effects on various aspects of life, perpetuating misunderstandings, and barriers to treatment. It is one of the leading causes of years lost to disability worldwide [1].

The patients typically present to the hospital with the complains such as hallucinations, delusions and disorders of thought perception and implementation, stunted emotional expression, overall diminished zeal to concentrate and accomplish goals, troubled relationships, motor, and cognitive impairments.

While the clinical symptoms—such as hallucinations and delusions—are often the focus of treatment, understanding the quality of life (QoL) for individuals experiencing psychosis is crucial for holistic care [2].

This chapter explores the multifaceted aspects of QoL in the context of psychosis, examining its definitions, determinants, impacts, and potential interventions.

2. Types of psychosis

Psychosis is a composite of several psychological symptoms leading to loss of contact with reality.

2.1 Causes of primary psychosis

1. *Schizophrenia*: A chronic condition that often involves hallucinations, delusions, and cognitive impairments.

2. *Schizoaffective disorder*: A combination of symptoms of schizophrenia and mood disorder symptoms such as depression or mania.

3. *Brief reactive psychotic disorder*: Characterized by sudden, short-term psychotic episodes, often triggered by stress or trauma.

4. *Substance-induced psychotic disorder*: Results from the use of drugs, including alcohol, hallucinogens, or withdrawal from substances.

5. *Psychotic disorders due to medical conditions*: Psychosis arising from neurological diseases, infections, or other medical conditions.

6. *Cycloid psychosis*: An acute form of psychosis with psychotic and mood symptoms that progress quickly [3].

2.2 Causes of secondary psychosis

1. *Congenital disorders*—For example, velocardiofacial syndrome or agenesis of corpus callosum.

2. *Toxic or substance-induced disorders*: Poisoning from lead, mercury, arsenic, PCP, MDMA, LSD, cannabis, or alcohol.

3. *Drug induced*—For example, the use of drugs like antimalarials, steroids, or isoniazid.

4. *Cerebrovascular disorders*—Such as stroke or subdural hematomas.

5. *Secondary to a disease condition*—For example, psychosis associated with temporal lobe epilepsy, N-methyl D-aspartate (NMDA) receptor encephalitis [3].

3. Etiology of psychosis

Onset of psychosis may be a result of a primary psychiatric disorder/s, illicit substance use, and another neurologic or medical condition. Several brain abnormalities have been implicated with the onset of psychotic disorders, including reduced gray matter volume particularly in the prefrontal, superior, and medial temporal lobes (**Figure 1**) [5].

In comparison with ventricle size of the normal brain, the ventricular size of the patient with schizophrenia is increased (**Figure 2**).

Primary psychotic disorders are considered neurodevelopmental abnormalities and are hypothesized to develop in utero, although the manifestations of full-blown psychosis occurs only after exposure to epigenetic and/or environmental risk factors such as substance abuse, stress, immigration, infection, postpartum period, or other medical causes. There is a considerable evidence for the association of genetic risk factors in the pathogenesis of psychotic disorders [5].

The etiology of psychosis is complex and multifactorial, involving a combination of biological, psychological, and environmental factors.

3.1 Genetic factors

Presence of psychotic disorders in the family can increase the risk of developing psychotic disorders. The risk of development of schizophrenia further increases to 40% when both the parents have schizophrenia. The chances of development of

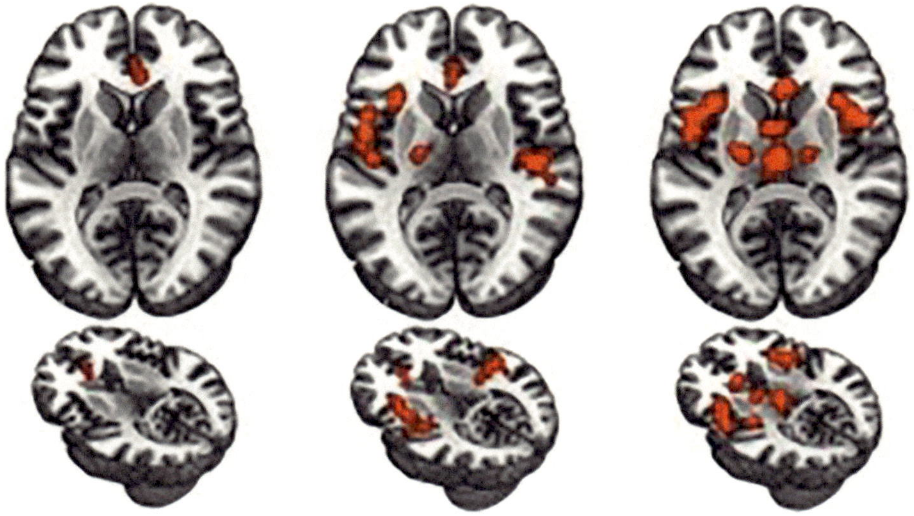

Figure 1.
Progression of gray matter damage in clinically high-risk patients, recently diagnosed patients of schizophrenia and chronic schizophrenia (left to right) [4].

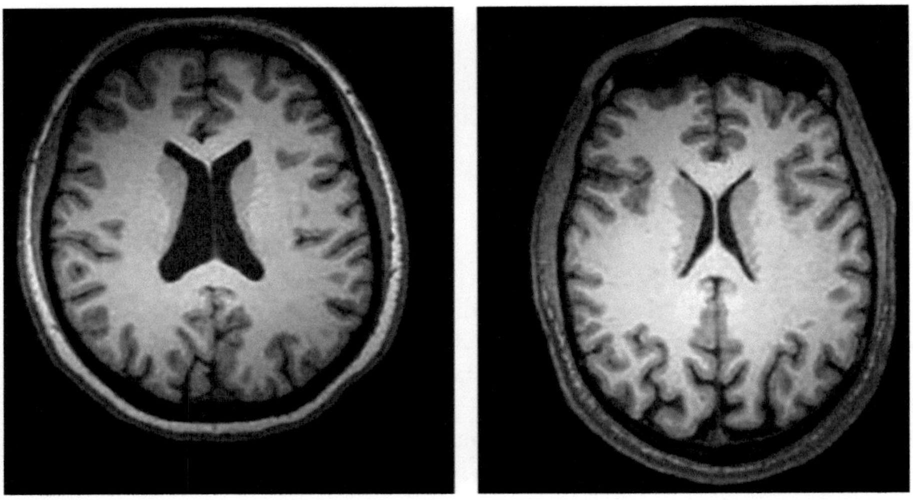

Figure 2.
Ventricles in the patient of Schizophrenia (left) with the ventricles of a normal person (right) [6].

psychosis can be as high as 60% in case of twins, whereas, in case of first-degree relatives, the risk of disease development is about 10%. Several reports of linkages of schizophrenia to loci on chromosomes 1,2,5,6,8,10,13,15,22 have been established. Recently, genes encoding for neuregulin-1, dysbindin, and D-amino acid oxidase have been identified [7].

3.2 Neurochemical factors

Imbalances in several neurotransmitters, particularly dopamine and serotonin in the brain, play a significant role in the etiopathogenesis of psychosis [7].

3.3 Brain structure

Several studies have identified irregularities in certain areas of the brain region including decreased gray matter volume (GMV), atypical cortical thickness in the prefrontal cortex, parietal lobes, and temporal lobes in the development of psychosis. Reduced cortical thickness in the corpus callosum, hippocampus, and posterior central gyrus has also been reported [8].

3.4 Environmental stressors

Environmental stressors including but not limited to fetal hypoxia in offsprings of parents with psychosis, experiencing bullying and childhood trauma, PTSD in war veterans, sexual assault victims, substance abuse, and significant life changes can trigger or exacerbate negative effects and severity of psychotic episodes [8].

3.5 Medical conditions

Certain medical illnesses affecting the brain such as infections, traumatic brain injuries, Alzheimer's disease, Lewy body dementia, advanced multiple sclerosis (MS), stroke, brain tumors, and viral encephalitis can lead to the development of psychotic symptoms [8].

4. Incidence and prevalence

Psychosis affects a person's thoughts, perceptions, and behaviors. It can cause people to lose touch with reality, experience hallucinations, and have delusions. The exact incidence and prevalence of psychosis can vary depending on the specific definition used and the population being studied.

As per the existing literature, the overall incidence of a first-time episode of psychosis and schizophrenia, as a specific subset of psychotic disorders, is approximately 50 in 100,000 people per year and 15 in 100,000 people per year, whereas the lifetime prevalence of psychosis and schizophrenia is estimated to be around 3% and 1%, respectively.

5. Symptomatology

Symptomatology of psychosis is characteristically described into two main types, that is, positive and negative symptoms.

5.1 Positive symptoms

Positive symptoms of psychosis add to or alter a person's thoughts, experiences of reality, often leading to a distorted perception of the world. These include:

1. *Hallucinations*: These involve sensing or perceiving things that are not present. Visual, tactile, and olfactory hallucinations although are present but auditory hallucinations are commonly observed.

2. *Delusions*: These are strong and fixated beliefs not amenable to change. Common delusions including delusion of paranoia (feeling persecuted) and delusion of grandiosity (feeling unusually powerful or important), and delusions of reference (believing that ordinary events have special meanings) are observed in people with psychosis.

3. *Disorganized thinking*: This can manifest as incoherent speech, difficulty organizing thoughts, or jumping between topics. It may also present as disorganized or erratic behavior that is inappropriate for the situation.

4. *Agitation or catatonia*: Some patients with psychosis may exhibit hyperactivity or restlessness, while others may become unresponsive or display unusual postures [9].

5.2 Negative symptoms

Negative symptoms refer to the absence or reduction of normal emotional responses or behaviors. These can significantly impact an individual's ability to function and engage with the world.

Key negative symptoms include:

1. *Affective flattening*: This involves a diminished emotional expression, leading to a lack of facial expressions, gestures, and eye contact.

2. *Avolition*: A lack of motivation or inability to initiate and persist in activities. This can manifest as neglect of personal hygiene or withdrawal from social interactions.

3. *Anhedonia*: A reduced ability to experience pleasure or interest in activities that were once enjoyable, leading to social withdrawal.

4. *Alogia*: This refers to poverty of speech, where the individual provides limited responses or shows reduced verbal communication.

5. *Social withdrawal*: Individuals may isolate themselves, withdrawing from friends, family, and social activities, contributing to a cycle of loneliness and worsening symptoms [9].

6. Defining quality of life

Quality of life (QOL) is a comprehensive and a holistic perception of overall physical, psychological, social, and material well-being which can be evaluated both individually and objectively. The World Health Organization (WHO) elaborates on the concept of quality of life as "the individual's perception of their position in life in the context of the culture and value systems in which they live and in relation to their goals."

The aspect of QOL is an important in the planning, assessment, and implementation of health services and guidelines for various long-term illnesses including the wide array of mental health disorders.

In healthcare, the QOL is assessed as the overall influence of health state on the well-being of the individual. The association assumes greater significance as various studies have highlighted poor QOL in patients suffering with several mental disorders such as schizophrenia, major depressive disorder, and bipolar disorders.

Psychosis is incapacitating illness, wherein the patients with demonstrate poor social skills, undesirable outcomes, and reduced overall functioning [10].

The patients tend to experience discontentment owing to depreciated working capacity, broken social construct, and a depreciated QOL by virtue of neurocognitive deficits along with patients' impoverished cognizance about their prevailing mental condition. The existing literature highlights the prodigal relationship among psychopathology, adverse symptoms, and poor QOL in patients during the course of their psychotic ailment [10].

Patients suffering with psychotic disorders experience a wide array of symptoms including but not limited to reduced concentration, reduced motivation, low or depressed mood, sleep disturbances, apprehensions, withdrawal from social settings, decline in operational capacity, disorganized thinking, hallucinations, and delusions, resulting in poor QOL. Most psychotic disorders are preceded by a prodromal phase in which a multitude of clinically high-risk (CHR) symptoms of psychosis, psychosocial deficits, and a reduction in self-related health occurs. This phase offers an excellent commencing point for reducing clinically high-risk (CHR) individuals of psychosis and, thereby, preventing transition to frank psychosis [10].

A recent study has highlighted that clinically high-risk states are characterized by consistent and prodigious impairments in QoL, when compared to healthy controls and people with other neurotic disorders [11].

A similar association among QoL and psychopathology and the severity of both positive and depressive symptoms in clinically high-risk patients has also been established, as predictors of poor QoL in CHR states. Anxiety states, cognitive deficiencies, and reduced functioning were also predictors of poor QoL in CHR states.

Common markers, that is, poor physical health and an overall unhealthy lifestyle, are predictors of ultra-high risk (UHR) patients and should be monitored regularly [12].

In recent community studies, the presence of psychotic symptoms was associated with poorer SRH. In the context of psychosis, QoL can be influenced by:

- *Physical health*: Chronic illnesses or side effects of medications can significantly impact daily functioning.
- *Psychological well-being*: Symptoms of psychosis can lead to feelings of distress, anxiety, and depression, further diminishing QoL.
- *Social relationships*: The stigma associated with mental illness can result in social isolation, affecting personal relationships and support systems.
- *Environmental factors*: Access to resources, safe housing, and supportive environments play a critical role in enhancing QoL.

7. Determinants of quality of life in psychosis

Several factors can influence QoL in individuals with psychosis:

1. *Severity of symptoms*: The intensity and frequency of psychotic episodes can directly affect an individual's ability to function in daily life.
2. *Coping mechanisms*: Adaptive coping strategies can mitigate the impact of psychosis on QoL, while maladaptive strategies may exacerbate difficulties.
3. *Social support*: Strong support networks can provide emotional assistance and practical help, improving overall QoL.
4. *Treatment engagement*: Active participation in treatment plans, including therapy and medication adherence, is associated with better QoL outcomes.
5. *Life events*: Stressful life events or changes in circumstances can have profound effects on mental health and perceived QoL [13].

Assessing the quality of life (QoL) in patients with psychosis is crucial for understanding the impact of the disorder and guiding treatment.

8. Several scales developed for this purpose, each focusing on different dimensions of QoL: Some commonly used scales are as follows

8.1 WHOQOL-BREF

It is a short version of the World Health Organization Quality of Life Assessment (WHOQOL), it evaluates QoL across four domains: physical health, psychological health, social relationships, and environment [14].

Use: Suitable for a wide range of populations, including those with mental health disorders.

8.2 Quality of life scale (QLS)

Description: Specifically designed for individuals with schizophrenia, the QLS assesses QoL through various domains, including interpersonal relationships, work, and leisure activities.

Use: Provides insight into the subjective experience of quality of life in psychosis [15].

8.3 EQ-5D

Description: A widely used generic instrument to measure health-related QoL. It assesses five dimensions: mobility, self-care, usual activities, pain/discomfort, and anxiety/depression.

Use: Can be used to comp are QoL across different health conditions, including psychosis [16].

9. Impact of psychosis

The effects of psychosis can be profound and far-reaching encompassing almost all the domains and aspects of one's life:

9.1 Impact on functioning

Both positive and negative symptoms can severely impact an individual's daily functioning, relationships, and overall quality of life. Positive symptoms may lead to misunderstandings, while negative symptoms can result in social isolation and a lack of motivation to engage in treatment or seek help [17].

Individuals may face challenges in maintaining relationships, employment, and self-care due to symptoms. Psychosis can deeply affect individuals on multiple levels, influencing their emotional, cognitive, and social functioning. Understanding these impacts is crucial for developing effective support systems and treatment strategies. Here are the key areas where psychosis can have a significant personal impact:

9.1.1 Social isolation

Social isolation is a key finding observed frequently in individuals with psychosis. Delusions of paranoia, that is, the fixated and falsified beliefs that others have harmful intentions toward them, have been observed to contribute to social withdrawal by furthering social anxiety or threat, particularly in those with a psychotic disorder or an increased predisposition for frank psychosis [18].

If paranoid delusions are eminent in social gatherings, the individual tends to distinguish it as threatful stimuli, which tends to impact the vigor to partake in social obligations, and ultimately, the person retracts from the society as a precautionary measure and if the perceived threat and distress decreases on withdrawal, the retractable behavior is reinforced [18].

While such a retracting behavior might feel rewarding at first, a socially isolated person is incapable to review set paranoid beliefs based on positive social interactions.

With continuous social isolation periods may work to exacerbate the delusions of paranoia, which could snowball in to a cycle of social exclusion.

The existing literature suggests that social isolation is a prominent adversary for deteriorating physical health, episodes of psychotic relapse/s, retractions from interpersonal/social interactions accompanied by feelings of disinterest, and unconcerned attitude [19].

These findings reiterate the bio-ecosystem theory of negative symptoms that explain the impact of several socio-cultural factors' environmental factors on negative symptoms and psychosis relapse [20].

It remains to be elucidated whether social withdrawal is a prelude to psychosis relapse or a consequence of the illness itself.

Social withdrawal, in all its manifestations, could therefore be an intervention target of choice after a psychotic episode to break vicious cycles of avoidance and potentially prevent reoccurrence of symptoms.

9.1.2 Stigma and discrimination

Individuals may face societal stigma, making it harder to connect with others and leading to feelings of loneliness. Social stigma in people with psychosis has garnered substantial attention owing to the undesirable influences in several spheres of life.

Social stigma affects disease awareness, management, and adherence to drug treatment.

People with psychosis tend to anticipate and corroborate the rejection by the society and incorporate the ostracizing views into their own thought processes, leading to self-stigmatization, which occurs frequently in the lives of people suffering with psychosis and their families.

This often works as an impediment to recovery from the disease process and the accomplishment of life goals [21].

9.2 Occupational challenges

9.2.1 Difficulty in maintaining employment

Cognitive impairments combined with the unpredictability of symptom onset can make it challenging to keep a job or perform at the same level. An extensive body of research recognizes social stigma due to psychosis as a significant barrier to employability in people living with serious mental health conditions. Several studies have highlighted that people with mental illnesses were subject to discrimination, while recruitments, ill-suited behaviors, and generalized prejudice post disclosure of mental health problems in the workplace [22].

9.2.2 Career limitations

Individuals may feel forced to change career paths or reduce work hours, impacting financial stability and personal fulfillment.

Psychosis is ranked by WHO as the ninth most disabling condition. Career disruptions are extensively observed among people with psychosis. Even in the people who attain jobs, the length of employment is generally very short, in some cases lasting less than 1 year. According to a survey of people with psychotic disorders, only about 14% of people with psychotic disorders maintained the employment for 6 months or more. Patients who lose their jobs lack an integrated social life, improved symptom level, good quality of life, and better self-esteem, with long-term unemployment being a plausible consequence. The overall outcomes of job insecurity, with the limited intra-personal and inter-personal associations, accrue to loss of function and an overall poor quality of life [23].

It can be emphasized that disabilities due to the psychotic disorders are a prelude to layoffs from paid employment from almost all types of establishments. Patients with psychotic disorders are not only denied the choice in employment spheres, but also face stigma, discrimination, monetary disadvantages, and loss of health benefits. Up to 70 percent of people with severe mental illness express a desire to work [24].

9.3 Psychological effects

9.3.1 Distress and anxiety

The experience of hallucinations or delusions can be terrifying, contributing to the already existing angst, leaving the individual anxious and distraught. The negative connotation exists over the gamut of subclinical and clinical expression of psychopathology, though the association is robust in the clinical range.

The symptoms and syndromes of anxiety are mostly present in majority of the patients with psychosis, and these affective symptoms help distinguish and delineate various diverse subgroups within the individuals with psychotic illness.

Thus, affective deregulations (anxiety, depression, and outbursts of anger and rapid mood swings) and distortions are expressed alongside a range of psychotic disorders, which may be thought off as a result of altered mentation that casts an impact on each other, for example, affective dysregulation giving rise to psychotic symptoms [25].

9.3.2 Depression

Individuals suffering from psychotic depression may experience feelings of hopelessness or sadness, especially if they struggle with the realities of their condition or face stigma.

Depression as a sequel to psychosis may largely orbit around individuals' altered perceptions of reality around their own identity. Similarly, one might expect the psychological reaction to current, ongoing positive symptoms in the acute episode to be important.

A person suffering with depression tends to gloomy and despondent for most part of the day, and there is a loss of excitement and enthusiasm for the activities that the person enjoyed earlier [25].

Although independently depression has a significant risk on the health, longevity, and unemployment contributing to poor outcomes in terms quality of life of the patient, it assumes greater significance in situations where it co-exists with psychotic disorders.

The coexistence of depression with schizophrenia is important, because it is conspicuously associated with increased suicidality. As the International Suicide Prevention Trial, suicidal behavior and ideations in people with psychotic disorders were described as 'a seriously under-treated life-threatening condition.'

According to a study, relapse into the illness is recurrent and the total duration of in-patient treatment is longer in those with significant depression.

9.3.3 Loss of self-esteem

Psychotic episodes can be challenging by questioning one's sense of identity, leading them to feel unsure or inhibited. A low level of self-esteem often accompanies psychosis along with specific symptoms, such as hallucinations and persecutory delusions [26].

Several studies have affirmed a robust association of negative self-esteem with positive symptoms. Reduced self-worth is related to paranoia, one of the cardinal features in psychosis. Individuals who demonstrate paranoid reactions tend to experience fear of being intentionally harmed by others to a higher degree compared to other individuals.

In people with psychotic disorders, negative self-esteem can be strongly influenced by social stress. Stress sensitization may play a pivotal role in this process. Stress sensitization may develop when people with psychosis are constantly exposed to the environmental risk factor(s) and these individuals tend to exhibit greater psychological and/or physiological response to stress over time.

The presence of low self-esteem among individuals with psychotic disorders is a well-documented and is a contributing factor in the formation of psychotic symptoms.

Negative self-evaluation is connected to the severity and maintenance of delusions and hallucinations, suicidal ideations, more relapses, and poor quality of life.

Research has highlighted that patients with psychotic disorders tend to have dented personal and professional relationships specifically owing to the negative self-beliefs leading to higher distress at the onset of illness [27].

9.4 Cognitive effects

Cognitive impairment is universally encountered in primary psychotic disorders, with approximately 80% of patients exhibiting clinically significant impairment.

Some studies have claimed that even in the absence of clinically significant cognitive impairment, all the affected individuals with a primary psychotic disorder perform at a level subpar to what would be expected had they never developed a psychotic illness. The available evidence does suggest that cognitive impairment is common, with one study reporting clinically significant impairment in up to 60% of patients with psychoses.

The decline in the cognitive performance tends to be somewhat larger for the tests that assess memory, processing speed, and verbal fluency with the largest patient-control differences observed for tests of attention and learning, whereas the decline is insignificant for measures of language and vocabulary and spatial reasoning [28].

This cognitive decline tends to hamper functioning in routine tasks such as cooking, cleaning, and managing finances thereby mandating the need for assistance to navigate through day-to-day life.

9.4.1 Impaired thought processes

Disorganized and derailed thinking, tangentiality, and circumstantiality, that is, moving from one point in the argument to the other with excessive and unnecessary details, inventing words that have no meaning and difficulty in concentrating on tasks can thwart overall decision-making and problem-solving abilities required for the day-to-day activities. Challenges with short-term memory, difficulty in recalling tasks or important information, and a lack of insight about the condition have been commonly observed in a significant number of patients leading to difficulty in recognizing the need for treatment and complicating recovery [29].

9.4.1.1 Delusions

Delusions, described as fixed, false beliefs not based on reality, are a common symptom observed in patients of psychosis. They can be very distressing for the person and tend to hamper the daily functioning. Several forms of delusions observed in the patients of psychosis are delusion of persecution, grandeur, reference, paranoid delusions, somatic delusions [30].

9.4.1.2 Hallucinations

Hallucinations are the sensory perceptions in the absence of any external stimulus. These are common feature of psychosis causing the person to be detached from reality. They can be visual, auditory, tactile, olfactory, or gustatory. Auditory hallucinations are most commonly observed in psychosis.

Other impairments including thought blocking, that is, the person's thoughts are suddenly interrupted or stopped, thought insertions, that is, the person believes that their thoughts are being inserted into their mind by an alien source, thought withdrawal, that is, the person believes that their thoughts are being taken out of their mind by an outside source, and thought broadcasting, that is, the person believes that their thoughts are being broadcast to others are observed in patients of psychosis.

Psychosocial stress is a potential contributing risk factor in the relapse of psychosis. Psychosocial stress can be described as emotional, physical, and psychological in response to social triggers. These stressors can be grouped as chronic (e.g., long-term unemployment), life events (e.g., homelessness), and minor daily hassles (e.g., offensive comments). A social stressor has been commonly reported to occur prior to an episode of psychosis, and a high number of stressful events have been commonly seen to precede the onset of frank psychosis. These findings are in line with the stress-vulnerability model, which states that collective exposure to psychosocial stressors is combined with bio-psychosocial vulnerability in the predisposed individuals to give rise to mental health difficulties.

Furthermore, high level of psychosocial stress has been observed in the individuals with psychosis compared to healthy individuals. In other words, patients with psychosis may present with heightened stress sensitivity and/or might be exposed to a higher number of stressful events compared to the healthy population [31].

9.5 Strained relationships

9.5.1 Withdrawal from relationships

Fear of being judged or misunderstood can cause individuals to withdraw from social circles including close relatives thereby acting as a harbinger of Psychosis. The support of the families are paramount for the patients with psychosis, in leading with a range of emotional, relational, and practical challenges. Families experience stress, confusion, anxiety of their own in providing additional support to the loved one with psychosis. The experience of psychosis is unsettling not only for the patients but influences family dynamics as well. The inability of family and friends may struggle to understand the plight of the patients with psychosis, which leads to misunderstandings and conflicts. Considering various constructs in the etiopathogenesis of psychotic disorders, emotional relationships, romantic or otherwise, have a pivotal role in reducing or exacerbating, psychotic experiences by addressing paranoid thoughts and behaviors. A companion or a close confidante may provide the indispensable emotional, practical, and financial support, which could increase resilience to stress [32].

9.6 Barriers to treatment

Reluctance to seek help: Stigmatization may discourage individuals from disclosing their symptoms and seeking treatment, fearing judgment or discrimination from healthcare providers.

Non- adherence to drug treatment: Cognitive decline and distortions in the patients of psychosis may lead to person to become skeptical about drug treatment, thereby affecting medication adherence and engagement in therapeutic interventions.

About one-third of the patients of psychosis are thought to be resistant to drug treatment, that is, sub-therapeutic plasma anti-psychotic levels chiefly attributed to poor drug adherence, which has been identified as one of the major causes for treatment failure.

Several factors have been implicated in complicating the treatment of psychosis including impact of symptoms on cognitive functions, absence of illness insight, stigma surrounding the illness, comorbid substance abuse, and social isolation. Although the number of patients on anti-psychotic drugs has increased over the years, insignificant progress has been made about improving medication adherence in these patients. Adherence difficulties complicate the clinical management for patients and eventually lead to poor treatment responses [33].

According to a study, a vast majority patients on various anti-psychotic drugs took their prescribed medication only for a brief time period (82%) of the prescribed antipsychotics that were consumed for a period of 3 months), indicating inadequate or under-treatment [34].

By underestimating non-adherence, prescribers may prematurely discontinue treatment, add concomitant medications, or increase dosages. Treatment failure in covert non-adherent individuals may lead to the faulty assumption of treatment resistance.

Recovery process: The journey to recovery can be arduous and nonlinear, with setbacks leading to frequent frustrations and discouragements, affecting motivation and hope for the future.

Lack of awareness: Many people have limited knowledge about psychosis, leading to misconceptions that it equates to violent behavior or an inability to function. This lack of understanding can foster fear and avoidance.

Stereotyping: Individuals with psychosis are often stereotyped as dangerous or unpredictable, which contributes to a culture of fear and discrimination.

10. Diagnosing psychosis

Diagnosing psychosis involves a comprehensive evaluation by a trained mental health care professional, on several parameters including:

- *Clinical interviews*: These remain the cornerstone in the diagnosis of psychosis to gather detailed personal and family history, symptoms, and functioning of the patient.

- *Mental status examinations*: A wide plethora of tests are employed in gaining an insight to the symptoms by assessing cognitive functioning, mood, memory, thought processes, and behavior.

- *Diagnostic criteria*: The diagnosis can be confirmed by integrating established criteria from the DSM-5 (Diagnostic and Statistical Manual of Mental Disorders) or ICD-10 (International Classification of Diseases) to identify specific disorders.

11. Treatment approaches

Effective treatment often requires a combination of pharmacological and psychosocial interventions:

- *Antipsychotic medications*: These are typically used to manage positive symptoms, helping to reduce hallucinations and delusions. They can be categorized into first-generation (typical) and second-generation (atypical) antipsychotics (**Table 1**).

- *Mood stabilizers and antidepressants*: Sometimes prescribed in cases where mood disorders are present.

- *Psychotherapy*: Cognitive behavioral therapy (CBT) can be effective in addressing distorted thinking and developing coping strategies for both positive and negative symptoms.

- *Cognitive behavioral therapy (CBT)*: Helps individuals identify and challenge distorted thoughts and beliefs.

- *Supportive therapy*: Provides emotional support and guidance through the recovery process. Social skills training, vocational rehabilitation, and support groups can help individuals rebuild their lives and improve their social functioning.

- *Family therapy*: Engages family members to improve communication and support within the family system.

- *Family involvement*: Educating family members about the condition and involving them in treatment can provide essential support for the individual [35].

Medication	Brand name	Dose	Half-life (hours)	Side effects
First-generation anti-psychotics				
Chlorpromazine	Thorazine	30–75 mg 2–4 times a day	23–37 h	Heart rate irregularities, allergic reactions, increased prolactin levels
Fluphenazine	Prolixin	2.5–10 mg 3–4 times a day	14–16 h	Muscle aches, neck spasms, drowsiness
Haloperidol	Haldol	0.5–2 mg 2–3 times a day	14–37 h	Hypotension, constipation, blurring of vision, insomnia
Pimozide	Orap	1–2 mg 4 times a day	55 h	akinesia, hyperhidrosis, somnolence
Sulpiride	Dogmatil	400–600 mg 2 times a day	8 h	Akathisia, drug-induced parkinsonism, hyperprolactinemia, tardive dyskinesia
Perphenazine	Trilafon	8–16 mg 2–4 times a day	9–12 h	Dizziness, blurring of vision, shuffling walk
Second-generation anti-psychotic drugs				
Aripiprazole	Abilify	40 mg 12 twice a day	75 h	Akathisia, resting tremor, shuffling gait, oculogyric crisis, hyper-prolactinemia
Asenapine	Saphris	2.5–10 mg twice a day	1.5 h	Somnolence, EPS (dystonia, akathisia), hyperglycemia
Brexpiprazole	Rexulti	2–4 mg four times a day	91 h	Weight gain, agitation, distress, trouble walking
Cariprazine	Vraylar	1.5 mg once a day	69 h	Sedation, fatigue, dizziness, akathisia
Clozapine	Clozaril	12.5 mg 1–2 times a day.	4–12 h	Blurring of vision, confusion, sweating, sleep disturbances
Iloperidone	Fanapt	12–24 mg twice a day.	18 h	Irregular heartbeat, difficulty in breathing, body ache
Lurasidone	Tracleer	40 mg four times a day.	20–40 h	Weight gain, akathisia, drug-induced parkinsonism
Olanzapine	Zyprexa	5–10 mg once a day.	21–59 h	Weight gain, somnolence, hyper-prolactinemia, hyper-triglyceridemia
Paliperidone	Invega	3 mg once a day.	24 h	Hypotension, uncontrolled muscle movements, shortness of breath
Quetiapine	Seroquel	50 mg once to thrice a day.	7 h	Drowsiness, dizziness, weight gain, postural hypotension
Risperidone	Risperdal	2 mg 1–2 times a day.	20 h	Drowsiness, parkinsonism, blurring of vision, akathisia
Ziprasidone	Geodon	40 mg twice a day.	10 h	Headache, restlessness, muscle cramps, decreased libido

Table 1.
List of drugs approved in the management of psychotic disorders.

Author details

Shreshth Khanna
Department of Pharmacology, Hamdard Institute of Medical Sciences and Research, Jamia Hamdard, New Delhi, India

*Address all correspondence to: shreshthkhanna@gmail.com

References

[1] Stuart H. Reducing the stigma of mental illness. Global Mental Health (Camb). 2016;**10**(3):e17

[2] Hurmuz M, Frandes M, Panfil A-L, Stoica I-P, Bredicean C, Giurgi-Oncu C, et al. Quality of life in patients with chronic psychotic disorders: A practical model for interventions in Romanian mental health centers. Medicina. 2022;**58**(5):615

[3] Maj M, van Os J, De Hert M, Gaebel W, Galderisi S, Green MF. The clinical characterization of the patient with primary psychosis aimed at personalization of management. World Psychiatry. 2021;**20**(1):4-33

[4] Liloia D, Brasso C, Cauda F. Updating and characterizing neuroanatomical markers in high-risk subjects, recently diagnosed and chronic patients with schizophrenia: A revised coordinate-based meta-analysis. Neuroscience & Biobehavioral Reviews. 2021;**123**:83-103

[5] Jia X, Wang J, Jiang W. Common gray matter loss in the frontal cortex in patients with methamphetamine-associated psychosis and schizophrenia. 2022;**36**:1-10

[6] Tyagi A, Singh V, Gore M. An efficient automated detection of schizophrenia using k-NN and bag of words features. SN Computer Science. 2023;**4**:1-10

[7] Chu T, Liu Y. An integrated genomic analysis of gene-function correlation on schizophrenia susceptibility genes. Journal of Human Genetics. 2010;**55**:285-292

[8] Crespo-Facorro B, Roiz-Santianez R, Perez-Iglesias R. Global and regional cortical thinning in first-episode psychosis patients: Relationships with clinical and cognitive features. Psychological Medicine. 2011;**41**:1449-1460

[9] Millan MJ, Fone K, Steckler T. Negative symptoms of schizophrenia: Clinical characteristics, pathophysiological substrates, experimental models and prospects for improved treatment. European Neuropsychopharmacology. 2014;**24**(5):645-692

[10] Michel C, Schmidt SJ, Schnyder N, et al. Associations of psychosis-risk symptoms with quality of life and self-rated health in the community. European Psychiatry. 2019;**62**:116-123

[11] Tsai CL, Chu CM, Lane HY. The comparison of lifestyles, mental risks, and physical indices among individuals with ultra-high risk of psychosis, patients with schizophrenia, and the general public. Behavioral Sciences (Basel). 2024;**14**(5):395

[12] Correll CU, Schooler NR. Negative symptoms in schizophrenia: A review and clinical guide for recognition, assessment, and treatment. Neuropsychiatric Disease and Treatment. 2020;**16**:519-534

[13] García-Fernández L, Romero-Ferreiro V, Sánchez-Pastor L. Impact of negative symptoms on functioning and quality of life in first psychotic episodes of schizophrenia. Journal of Clinical Medicine. 2022;**11**(4):983

[14] Kruithof N, Haagsma JA, Karabatzakis M. Validation and reliability of the Abbreviated World Health Organization Quality of Life Instrument (WHOQOL-BREF) in the

hospitalized trauma population. Injury. 2018;**49**(10):1796-1804

[15] Schaefer J, Giangrande E, Weinberger DR, Dickinson D. The global cognitive impairment in schizophrenia: Consistent over decades and around the world. Schizophrenia Research. 2013;**150**(1):42-50

[16] Winkler K, Lincoln TM, Wiesjahn M. How does loneliness interact with positive, negative and depressive symptoms of psychosis? New insights from a longitudinal therapy process study. Schizophrenia. 2024;**271**:179-185

[17] Ünal B, Akgül Ö, Binbay T. Association of wider social environment with relapse in schizophrenia: Registry based six-year follow-up study. Noropsikiyatri Arsivi. 2019;**56**:235-242

[18] Macias C, DeCarlo LT, Wang Q, Frey J, Barreira P, et al. Work interest as a predictor of competitive employment: Policy implications for psychiatric rehabilitation. Administration and Policy in Mental Health. 2001;**28**(4):279-297

[19] Eack SM, Newhill CE. Psychiatric symptoms and quality of life in schizophrenia: A meta-analysis. Schizophrenia Bulletin. 2007;**33**(5):1225-1237

[20] Vahedi S. World Health Organization Quality-of-Life Scale (WHOQOL-BREF): Analyses of their item response theory properties based on the graded responses model. Iranian Journal of Psychiatry. 2010;**5**(4):140-153

[21] Morese R, Palermo S, Torello C, Sechi F. Social Withdrawal and Mental Health: An Interdisciplinary Approach. London, UK: IntechOpen; 2020

[22] Phillips L, Francey S, Edwards J, McMurray N. Strategies used by psychotic individuals to cope with life stress and symptoms of illness: A systematic review. Anxiety, Stress, and Coping. 2009;**22**:371-410

[23] Chafi YK, Amare T, Haile K, Damene W, Tesfaye G, Minichil W. Prevalence and correlates of job loss among schizophrenia outpatients at St. AmanuelMental Specialized Hospital, Addis Ababa, Ethiopia; cross sectional study. PLoS One. 2020;**15**(12):e0242352

[24] MacKenzie MB, Abbott KA, Kocovski NL. Mindfulness-based cognitive therapy in patients with depression: Current perspectives. Neuropsychiatric Disease and Treatment. 2018;**14**:1599-1605

[25] Maximo JO, Nelson EA, Armstrong WP. Duration of untreated psychosis correlates with brain connectivity and morphology in medication-naive patients with first-episode psychosis. Biological Psychiatry: Cognitive Neuroscience and Neuroimaging. 2020;**5**(2):231-238

[26] Atherton S, Antley A, Evans N, Cernis E, Lister R, Dunn G, et al. Self-confidence and paranoia: An experimental study using an immersive virtual reality social situation. Behavioural and Cognitive Psychotherapy. 2016;**44**(1):56-64

[27] Tan EJ, Neill E, Rossell SL. Assessing the relationship between semantic processing and thought disorder symptoms in schizophrenia. Journal of the International Neuropsychological Society. 2015;**21**(8):629-638

[28] Berry N, Peters S, Haddock G, et al. How individuals with psychosis develop and maintain resilience to suicidal experiences through psychological

therapy: A qualitative study. BMC Psychiatry. 2024;**24**:874

[29] Moradell A, Casajús JA, Moreno LA, Vicente-Rodríguez G. Perspectives on diet and exercise interaction for healthy aging: Opportunities to reduce malnutrition risk and optimize fitness. Nutrients. 2025;**17**(3):596

[30] Strauss GP. A bioecosystem theory of negative symptoms in schizophrenia. Frontiers in Psychiatry. 2021;**12**:655471

[31] Batic-Mujanovic O, Poric S, Pranjic N, Ramic E, Alibasic E, Karic E. Influence of unemployment on mental health of the working age population. Materia Socio-Medica. 2017;**29**(2):92-96

[32] Krüger RT. Psychotic disorders. In: Disorder-Specific Psychodrama Therapy in Theory and Practice. Psychodrama in Counselling, Coaching and Education. Vol. 4. Singapore: Springer; 2024. DOI: 10.1007/978-981-99-7508-2_9

[33] El Abdellati K, De Picker L, Morrens M. Antipsychotic treatment failure: A systematic review on risk factors and interventions for treatment adherence in psychosis. Frontiers in Neuroscience. 2020;**14**:531763

[34] Kim EY, Jang MH. The mediating effects of self-esteem and resilience on the relationship between internalized stigma and quality of life in people with schizophrenia. Asian Nursing Research. 2019;**13**:257-263

[35] Purba FD, Anggriani Y, Murtini T. EQ-5D-5L in schizophrenia: Differences between patients and nurses' reports. Health and Quality of Life Outcomes. 2021;**19**(1):240

Chapter 2

The Fog of Schizophrenia: Cognitive Impairments and Their Impact on Daily Life

Mihaela Fadgyas Stanculete and Octavia Capatina

Abstract

Cognitive impairments are a central feature of schizophrenia, encompassing deficits in attention, memory, executive function, and social cognition that significantly impact daily functioning and quality of life. These impairments often emerge early, preceding the onset of psychotic symptoms, and remain persistent over time, contributing to challenges in employment, social relationships, and independent living. Unlike positive symptoms, cognitive deficits are resistant to traditional antipsychotic treatments and strongly predict long-term functional outcomes. The interplay between cognitive deficits and negative symptoms, such as apathy and social withdrawal, creates a cycle of dysfunction that exacerbates social and occupational impairments. Neurobiological mechanisms, including dysfunctions in the prefrontal cortex, hippocampus, and neurotransmitter systems such as dopamine, glutamate, and serotonin, underlie these deficits, further complicating their management. Cognitive remediation has emerged as a promising intervention, utilizing targeted training to improve cognitive performance and functional outcomes. By addressing cognitive dysfunction alongside pharmacological treatments and comprehensive approaches, cognitive remediation offers hope for enhancing the daily lives of individuals with schizophrenia. This manuscript explores the nature of cognitive deficits in schizophrenia, their interaction with other symptoms, long-term implications, and the potential of cognitive remediation as an effective therapeutic strategy.

Keywords: cognitive deficits, cognitive remediation, functional outcomes, neurobiology, schizophrenia

1. Introduction

Schizophrenia is a severe mental disorder that affects millions worldwide, characterized by disruptions in thought processes, emotional regulation, perception, and behavior. While symptoms such as hallucinations and delusions—the positive symptoms—are often the most recognizable, cognitive deficits are increasingly recognized as a central and persistent feature of the disorder. These impairments, spanning domains like attention, memory, executive functioning, and social cognition, are particularly debilitating, as they significantly impact functional outcomes such as employment, social relationships, and independent living. Unlike positive symptoms, which can fluctuate and respond well to antipsychotic treatments, cognitive deficits are stable, pervasive, and resistant to conventional therapies.

Emerging research highlights the interplay between cognitive deficits and other symptom domains, including the negative symptoms of apathy and social withdrawal. This interaction creates a cycle of dysfunction that compounds challenges in daily life. Neurobiological studies further implicate disruptions in brain regions such as the prefrontal cortex and hippocampus, as well as dysregulation in neurotransmitter systems like dopamine, glutamate, and serotonin, as underlying mechanisms of these deficits.

This chapter explores the multifaceted nature of cognitive impairments in schizophrenia, examining their neurobiological underpinnings, their interactions with other symptoms, and their implications for daily functioning and long-term outcomes. It also reviews promising interventions, particularly cognitive remediation, which aim to mitigate these deficits and enhance the quality of life for individuals with schizophrenia. By addressing these often-overlooked challenges, this chapter contributes to a broader understanding of the disorder and its impact.

2. Living through the fog: A clinical illustration of cognitive deficits

Maria, a 29-year-old graduate student, had always been a determined and talented scholar. But as she progressed through her studies, her life began to unravel in ways she could not fully understand. What started as small lapses in concentration gradually spiraled into profound cognitive challenges that overtook every aspect of her life.

During what should have been a routine day working on her research, Mary found herself unable to focus. Her thoughts, once clear and methodical, became fragmented and incoherent. The words on the page blurred together, and she struggled to comprehend even the simplest passages. Her memory failed her frequently; she would forget why she had walked into a room or lose track of her train of thought mid-sentence.

As these difficulties deepened, Maria's ability to maintain her academic performance plummeted. She missed deadlines, failed to complete assignments, and avoided meetings with her professors out of embarrassment and fear. Socially, Maria became increasingly withdrawn. Conversations, once an effortless exchange of ideas, now felt like daunting puzzles. She often misunderstood others, struggled to keep track of the dialogue, and felt overwhelmed by her inability to connect. Gradually, she retreated from her friends and colleagues, isolating herself in the small apartment she could barely manage to maintain.

When Maria finally sought medical help, she was diagnosed with schizophrenia, a severe mental illness marked by psychosis, including delusions, hallucinations, and disorganized thinking. She struggled with fixed, false beliefs that eroded her sense of reality and led her to make decisions that alienated her from others. Her cognitive impairments compounded these issues, leaving her unable to process or organize information effectively. Tasks as simple as paying bills, attending appointments, or preparing meals became monumental challenges.

Maria's condition affected every facet of her life. She was forced to leave her graduate program, abandoning the career she had worked so hard to build. With no financial stability and a diminished support network, she faced economic hardship and increasing dependency on public assistance. Her mental health declined further, as feelings of shame and hopelessness took root.

Although Maria attempted to engage in treatment, the journey was fraught with difficulties. Side effects from medications were difficult to tolerate, and her cognitive impairments made it challenging to consistently follow through with therapy or routines meant to support her recovery. The fragmented support systems available to her were insufficient to address the complexity of her needs.

Maria's story exemplifies the profound impact of cognitive deficits on daily functioning and quality of life for individuals with schizophrenia. Her struggles with attention, memory, and executive functioning, coupled with social withdrawal and occupational challenges, reflect the cognitive and negative symptom interplay described in this chapter. These deficits, as highlighted in Maria's case, are resistant to traditional antipsychotic treatments but are precisely the target of cognitive remediation strategies.

Interventions such as *Cognitive Remediation Therapy (CRT)* and *Computerized Cognitive Remediation Therapy (CCRT)*, detailed in later sections and summarized in **Table 1** [1–10], could directly address Maria's challenges. For instance, CRT's structured cognitive exercises could improve her working memory and organizational skills, helping her regain some independence in daily activities like paying bills and managing appointments. Similarly, social cognition training could enhance her ability to interpret and engage in conversations, reducing her sense of isolation.

Integrating these cognitive remediation strategies into Maria's treatment plan, alongside pharmacological interventions and social support, could not only mitigate her cognitive deficits but also restore a sense of purpose and connection in her life. By demonstrating the real-world applications of these interventions, Maria's case highlights the importance of comprehensive, individualized approaches to treatment in schizophrenia.

3. The spectrum of cognitive impairments

Cognitive impairments are a hallmark of schizophrenia, significantly affecting various core cognitive domains. These impairments encompass memory (both short-term and working memory), attention and focus, executive functioning (including planning, problem-solving, and decision-making), and verbal and visual learning. Understanding these domains is crucial for developing effective interventions and improving the quality of life for individuals with schizophrenia.

3.1 Memory impairments

Memory deficits in schizophrenia are particularly pronounced in both short-term and working memory. Short-term memory refers to the ability to hold a small amount of information in an active state for a brief period while working memory involves the manipulation and processing of that information [11, 12]. Research indicates that individuals with schizophrenia often exhibit significant impairments in these areas, which can hinder their ability to learn new information and perform tasks that require the retention of information over short periods [12]. Studies have shown that working memory deficits are associated with dysfunction in the prefrontal cortex, a brain region critical for higher-order cognitive processes [13]. This dysfunction can lead to difficulties in tasks that require the integration of new information with existing knowledge, ultimately impacting daily functioning and social interactions [14]. Furthermore, impairments in memory are not only prevalent but can also be static, indicating a neurodevelopmental aspect to these deficits that may persist throughout the lifespan [15].

Cognitive remediation intervention	Description	Effects on cognitive function	Impact on functionality	References
Cognitive Remediation Therapy (CRT)	A structured program that includes cognitive drills and compensatory strategies to improve cognitive deficits such as attention, memory, and executive function.	Significant improvements in cognitive performance, particularly in attention and memory tasks.	Enhances daily living skills, social interactions, and occupational functioning.	Kubota et al. [1], Nuechterlein et al. [2], Deste et al. [3]
Computerized Cognitive Remediation Therapy (CCRT)	Utilizes computer-based exercises targeting specific cognitive deficits.	Shows improvements in attention and executive function, with some studies indicating enhanced verbal learning.	May lead to better performance in social and occupational settings.	Klojčnik and Vukman [4], Chong et al. [5]
Multicomponent interventions	Combines cognitive remediation with other therapies, such as Cognitive Behavioral Therapy (CBT) and pharmacological treatments.	Results in improvements in cognitive functioning and reduction in depressive symptoms.	Enhances overall functioning by addressing both cognitive and emotional aspects.	Wastler et al. [6], Dark [7]
Social cognition training	Focuses on improving social cognitive skills, such as emotion recognition and theory of mind.	Improves social cognition, which is linked to better social functioning and reduced negative symptoms.	Enhances interpersonal relationships and community engagement.	Fernández-Sotos et al. [8], Tan [9]
Aerobic exercise combined with cognitive training	Integrates physical exercise with cognitive remediation strategies.	Enhances cognitive performance and may improve mood and motivation.	Promotes better functional outcomes through improved cognitive and physical health.	Nuechterlein et al. [10]
Cognitive Behavioral Therapy for Cognitive Dysfunction (CBT-CD)	A therapeutic approach that combines cognitive remediation with CBT techniques.	Improves cognitive flexibility and coping strategies.	Enhances overall functioning by addressing cognitive deficits and emotional regulation.	Wastler et al. [6]

Table 1.
Cognitive remediation interventions and their effects in schizophrenia.

3.2 Attention and focus

Attention deficits are another core cognitive impairment in schizophrenia. Individuals with the disorder often struggle to maintain focus on tasks, leading to difficulties in processing information and completing activities that require sustained attention [16, 17]. These attentional deficits can manifest in various ways, including challenges in filtering out distractions and shifting attention between tasks [18]. Research utilizing neuropsychological assessments has demonstrated that attention impairments in schizophrenia can significantly affect performance on tasks that require vigilance and concentration [19]. The relationship between attention deficits and cognitive functioning is complex, as attention is foundational for effective memory processing and executive functioning [20]. Consequently, deficits in attention can exacerbate other cognitive impairments, creating a cascading effect that further hinders overall cognitive performance and functional outcomes [21].

3.3 Executive functioning

Executive functioning encompasses a range of cognitive processes, including planning, problem-solving, and decision-making. Deficits in executive functioning are prevalent in schizophrenia and are linked to impairments in the prefrontal cortex [22, 23]. These deficits can manifest as difficulties in organizing thoughts, setting goals, and adapting to new situations, which are essential skills for navigating daily life [24]. Research has shown that individuals with schizophrenia often exhibit impairments in tasks that require cognitive flexibility, such as the Wisconsin Card Sorting Test, which assesses the ability to shift strategies based on changing rules [22]. Additionally, executive dysfunction is associated with negative symptoms of schizophrenia, such as apathy and lack of motivation, further complicating the functional outcomes for individuals with the disorder [19]. Understanding the mechanisms underlying executive dysfunction is crucial for developing targeted cognitive remediation strategies that can help improve these skills and enhance overall functioning [25, 26].

3.4 Verbal and visual learning

Verbal and visual learning deficits are also significant cognitive impairments in schizophrenia. These deficits can affect an individual's ability to acquire and retain new information, impacting their educational and occupational achievements [27]. Studies have shown that individuals with schizophrenia often perform poorly on tasks that require verbal memory, such as recalling words or sentences, as well as on visual learning tasks that involve recognizing patterns or objects [28]. The relationship between verbal and visual learning deficits and cognitive functioning is critical, as these skills are essential for effective communication and social interaction [29]. Furthermore, impairments in these areas can hinder the ability to engage in meaningful relationships and participate in community activities, ultimately affecting the quality of life for individuals with schizophrenia [30].

4. Neuroanatomical modifications: A basis for cognitive deficits

The neurological underpinnings of schizophrenia are intricate and involve specific brain regions, neurochemical processes, and structural and functional changes. Understanding these elements is critical for elucidating the pathophysiology of the disorder and developing more effective treatment approaches. Key brain regions implicated in schizophrenia include the prefrontal cortex (PFC), hippocampus, and other interconnected areas, each contributing to the cognitive and behavioral symptoms observed in the disorder.

4.1 Prefrontal cortex (PFC)

The prefrontal cortex is essential for executive functions such as decision-making, planning, and working memory. Dysfunctions in the PFC are consistently linked to the cognitive deficits characteristic of schizophrenia [31, 32]. Neuroimaging studies reveal reduced activity and weakened connectivity in the PFC, correlating with deficits in cognitive control and task performance [32–34]. These impairments may result in difficulties filtering irrelevant information and maintaining focus, intensifying the cognitive challenges faced by individuals with the disorder [32].

4.2 Hippocampus

The hippocampus is central to memory formation and spatial navigation. Structural abnormalities, such as reduced hippocampal volume, have been consistently observed in individuals with schizophrenia [35, 36]. These alterations are thought to underlie common deficits in verbal learning and memory. Moreover, the hippocampus's connectivity with the PFC is critical for integrating new information with prior knowledge, and disruptions in this network can further compound cognitive impairments [35].

4.3 Other regions

Additional brain regions implicated in schizophrenia include the anterior cingulate cortex (ACC) and the striatum. The ACC is involved in error detection and cognitive flexibility, while the striatum plays a significant role in reward processing and motivation [31, 37]. Abnormalities in these areas are linked to negative symptoms such as apathy and reduced motivation, complicating the clinical profile and limiting functional outcomes for affected individuals [32, 38].

5. Neurobiological factors underpinning cognitive impairments in schizophrenia

Cognitive impairments in schizophrenia arise from complex interactions between various neurotransmitter systems and neurobiological factors. Beyond the established roles of dopamine, glutamate, and acetylcholine, recent research has highlighted the involvement of vascular endothelial growth factor (VEGF) and neuregulin 1 (NRG1) in the cognitive dysfunction associated with the disorder. These factors contribute to schizophrenia's pathogenesis through their roles in neurodevelopment, neuroplasticity, and neurotransmitter interactions.

5.1 Dopamine dysregulation

Dopamine remains central to schizophrenia's neurobiology. Dysregulated dopamine activity in the mesolimbic pathway contributes to positive symptoms, while reduced mesocortical activity is associated with cognitive deficits and negative symptoms [31, 32, 39]. The psychosis-inducing effects of amphetamines further support dopamine's critical role [32].

5.2 Glutamate and GABA

NMDA receptor hypofunction and GABAergic disruptions are implicated in cognitive deficits and neural instability. Glutamate and GABA interact with dopamine, amplifying the disorder's cognitive and behavioral symptoms [40–42].

5.3 Acetylcholine (ACh)

The cholinergic system, crucial for learning and memory, is associated with cognitive deficits and negative symptoms in schizophrenia. Dysregulated ACh signaling also interacts with dopamine pathways, suggesting therapeutic potential for targeting this system [43, 44].

5.4 Norepinephrine (NE)

Norepinephrine, vital for attention and stress regulation, is linked to cognitive and emotional symptoms. Its interactions with dopamine and serotonin systems underscore its relevance in schizophrenia's complex neurobiology [45].

5.5 Serotonin (5-HT)

Serotonin dysregulation, particularly involving the 5-HT2A receptor, contributes to cognitive deficits and negative symptoms. Atypical antipsychotics, which often target serotonin, have shown efficacy in mitigating these impairments [46–48].

6. Emerging neurobiological factors

6.1 Vascular endothelial growth factor (VEGF)

VEGF, a signaling protein essential for angiogenesis and neuroplasticity, has been implicated in schizophrenia's cognitive deficits.

6.1.1 Cognitive function

Studies report significantly lower VEGF serum levels in schizophrenia, correlating with reduced prefrontal cortex volume and impairments in executive function and memory [49, 50]. Decreased VEGF receptor-2 expression in the frontal cortex further underscores its role in cognitive health [51].

6.1.2 Neurodevelopmental role

VEGF dysregulation during critical developmental periods, such as prenatal hypoxia, may contribute to the structural and functional brain abnormalities observed in schizophrenia [52, 53].

6.2 Neuregulin 1 (NRG1)

NRG1, a signaling protein involved in synaptic plasticity and myelination, has been identified as a schizophrenia susceptibility gene [54].

6.2.1 Cognitive dysfunction

NRG1 is critical for GABAergic neurotransmission in the prefrontal cortex, and disruptions in its signaling contribute to impairments in working memory and executive function [55]. Animal models with altered NRG1 expression exhibit schizophrenia-like cognitive deficits [56].

NRG1 influences NMDA receptor function and interacts with dopamine pathways, further linking it to schizophrenia's cognitive and behavioral symptoms [56, 57].

VEGF and NRG1 both play pivotal roles in neurodevelopment and neuroplasticity, and their dysregulation may exacerbate the cognitive impairments seen in schizophrenia. Impaired VEGF signaling could amplify deficits associated with NRG1 dysfunction, creating a feedback loop that worsens cognitive decline [50, 53, 56]. Environmental factors such as prenatal stress or hypoxia further disrupt these pathways, highlighting their role in schizophrenia's pathogenesis [52].

7. Cognitive deficits in schizophrenia: Distinct challenges and interrelationships

7.1 Cognitive deficits as distinct challenges

Cognitive impairments in schizophrenia are characterized by deficits in several core domains, including working memory, attention, executive function, and social cognition. These deficits are often stable over time and may even precede the onset of psychotic symptoms [32, 58]. Unlike positive symptoms, which tend to fluctuate in severity and often respond well to antipsychotic treatment, cognitive deficits are more persistent and resistant to standard interventions [32].

Research has consistently shown that cognitive deficits are strong predictors of functional outcomes in schizophrenia, often surpassing the impact of positive symptoms [18, 59]. For example, individuals with significant cognitive impairments frequently face challenges in daily living, employment, and social relationships, contributing to a reduced quality of life [18, 59]. Addressing cognitive dysfunction is therefore critical in treatment plans, as improvements in cognitive function have the potential to enhance overall functioning and life satisfaction [59, 60].

7.2 Interrelationship with positive and negative symptoms

Although cognitive deficits are distinct from positive and negative symptoms, they are interrelated and influence each other in significant ways. Negative symptoms, such as apathy and lack of motivation, often mediate the relationship between cognitive dysfunction and social cognition, thereby affecting functional outcomes [59, 61]. For instance, severe negative symptoms can exacerbate cognitive impairments, leading to greater difficulties in social and occupational functioning [59, 61].

Positive symptoms, while more pronounced during acute episodes, also interact with cognitive deficits. Studies have found that positive symptoms, such as hallucinations and delusions, can impair cognitive performance, particularly in tasks requiring attention and working memory [60, 62]. Conversely, cognitive impairments may amplify the severity of positive symptoms by reducing the individual's ability to engage with reality, potentially leading to more pronounced hallucinations or delusions [63].

7.3 The role of neurobiological mechanisms

The neurobiological mechanisms underlying cognitive deficits, positive symptoms, and negative symptoms appear to differ, suggesting that distinct brain regions and neurotransmitter systems are involved. Cognitive impairments in schizophrenia have been linked to dysfunction in the prefrontal cortex and hippocampus, areas critical for memory and executive function [64, 65]. Positive symptoms, on the other hand, are primarily associated with dopaminergic dysregulation in the mesolimbic pathway, while negative symptoms are thought to involve disruptions in the mesocortical pathway [32, 66].

Neurochemical factors also play a role in cognitive dysfunction. Alterations in glutamate and serotonin signaling have been implicated, further complicating the interplay between cognitive deficits and other symptom domains [67]. Understanding these neurobiological distinctions is crucial for developing targeted interventions that address the unique challenges posed by cognitive deficits and their interactions with positive and negative symptoms.

8. Cognitive deficits and daily functioning in schizophrenia

8.1 Cognitive deficits and functional outcomes

Cognitive impairments in schizophrenia, including deficits in attention, memory, and executive functioning, are critical predictors of functional outcomes. These impairments often hinder daily living activities, such as managing finances, maintaining employment, and fostering social relationships [68, 69]. Research by Sheffield et al. demonstrated a strong link between cognitive performance and real-world functionality, highlighting that individuals with poor cognitive ability show diminished capacities across interpersonal, occupational, and community domains [68]. These findings underscore the need to address cognitive deficits in treatment plans to improve functionality and overall quality of life.

8.2 Interplay with positive and negative symptoms

The relationship between cognitive deficits and other symptom domains, particularly negative symptoms, further complicates their impact on functionality. Negative symptoms, such as apathy, lack of motivation, and social withdrawal, exacerbate cognitive impairments, creating a cycle of dysfunction that hinders daily activities [58]. Du's research suggests that negative symptoms mediate the relationship between cognitive deficits and functional outcomes, emphasizing that targeting these symptoms could improve cognitive performance and enhance functionality [58]. Similarly, positive symptoms like hallucinations and delusions can interfere with cognitive processes, particularly in tasks requiring attention and working memory, further impacting functional capacity [60, 62]. This interplay highlights the need for comprehensive treatment approaches that address all symptom domains to optimize recovery.

8.3 Long-term functional implications

Cognitive deficits in schizophrenia often emerge early and may worsen over time, leading to profound long-term functional impairments [70, 71]. These deficits can precede the onset of psychosis by nearly a decade, indicating that early cognitive decline is a hallmark of the disorder [70]. This early onset affects critical milestones, such as educational attainment and career development, ultimately reducing independence and quality of life [71].

McCleery and Nuechterlein emphasize that cognitive impairment is one of the strongest determinants of community functioning in individuals with psychotic disorders, with persistent cognitive deficits leading to challenges in engaging in meaningful activities, increased social isolation, and a diminished quality of life [71]. Addressing these deficits early and effectively is crucial for mitigating their long-term impact on individuals' daily lives and societal integration.

8.4 Cognitive remediation and functional improvement

Given the profound influence of cognitive deficits on functionality, cognitive remediation has emerged as a promising intervention. This approach involves targeted training and rehabilitation aimed at enhancing specific cognitive domains, such as attention, memory, and executive functioning [64, 71]. Research has demonstrated that cognitive remediation can improve cognitive performance and lead to better functional outcomes in daily life. For example, Barlati et al. and Charernboon found that structured cognitive training significantly enhanced individuals' ability to manage daily tasks, maintain employment, and engage socially [64, 71].

Moreover, Wu et al. underscored the importance of combining cognitive remediation with novel psychopharmacological interventions to address cognitive dysfunction comprehensively. This integrated approach has the potential to improve both cognitive functioning and overall quality of life in individuals with schizophrenia [70].

To further illustrate the potential of cognitive remediation in addressing the multifaceted cognitive deficits in schizophrenia, **Table 1** summarizes various cognitive remediation interventions. Each intervention's description, targeted cognitive domains and impact on functionality are outlined, providing a clear comparison of their efficacy.

9. Conclusions

The metaphor of "fog" aptly describes the disorienting and pervasive impact of neurocognitive impairments in schizophrenia. These deficits, which span multiple cognitive domains, are not only widespread but also severe, profoundly affecting daily functioning and diminishing quality of life. Understanding the neurobiological underpinnings and the complex interplay between cognitive deficits and other symptoms is critical for developing effective interventions. By targeting these impairments, it may be possible to lift the cognitive fog, improving clarity of thought and fostering better outcomes for individuals living with schizophrenia.

Acknowledgements

The author acknowledges the use of ChatGPT for language polishing of the manuscript.

Conflict of interest

The authors declare no conflict of interest.

Author details

Mihaela Fadgyas Stanculete* and Octavia Capatina
Department of Neuroscience, Psychiatry, University of Medicine and Pharmacy Iuliu Hatieganu Cluj Napoca, Romania

*Address all correspondence to: mihaela.fadgyas@umfcluj.ro

References

[1] Kubota R, Ikezawa S, Oi H, Oba MS, Izumi S, Tsuno R, et al. Valuable interaction with cognitive remediation and optimal antipsychotics for recovery in schizophrenia (VICTORY-S): Study protocol for an interventional, open-label, randomized comparison of combined treatment with cognitive remediation and lurasidone or paliperidone. Frontiers in Psychiatry. 2024;**14**:1331356. DOI: 10.3389/fpsyt.2023.1331356

[2] Nuechterlein KH, Ventura J, Subotnik KL, Gretchen-Doorly D, Turner LR, Casaus LR, et al. A randomized controlled trial of cognitive remediation and long-acting injectable risperidone after a first episode of schizophrenia: Improving cognition and work/school functioning. Psychological Medicine. 2020;**52**(8):1517-1526. DOI: 10.1017/s0033291720003335

[3] Deste G, Barlati S, Galluzzo A, Corsini P, Valsecchi P, Turrina C, et al. Effectiveness of cognitive remediation in early versus chronic schizophrenia: A preliminary report. Frontiers in Psychiatry. 2019;**10**:236. DOI: 10.3389/fpsyt.2019.00236

[4] Klojčnik M, Vukman KB. The effectiveness of computerized cognitive remediation therapy (CCRT) for deficits in attention and executive functions in depression: A pilot study. Applied Neuropsychology. Adult. 2021;**30**(3):306-314. DOI: 10.1080/23279095.2021.1941965

[5] Chong NIM, Maniam Y, Chua YC, Tang C. The implementation and review of cognitive remediation training for first episode psychosis in Singapore. Frontiers in Psychiatry. 2021;**12**:784935. DOI: 10.3389/fpsyt.2021.784935

[6] Wastler HM, Moe AM, Pine JG, Breitborde NJK. Cognition and suicide risk among individuals with first-episode psychosis: A 6-month follow-up. Psychiatric Rehabilitation Journal. 2022;**45**(1):27-33. DOI: 10.1037/prj0000488

[7] Dark F, Galloway G, Gray M, Cella M, De Monte V, Gore-Jones V, et al. Reward learning as a potential mechanism for improvement in schizophrenia spectrum disorders following cognitive remediation: Protocol for a clinical, nonrandomized, pre-post pilot study. JMIR Research Protocols. 2024;**13**:e52505. DOI: 10.2196/52505

[8] Fernández-Sotos P, Torío I, Fernández-Caballero A, Navarro E, González P, Dompablo M, et al. Social cognition remediation interventions: A systematic mapping review. PLoS One. 2019;**14**(6):e0218720. DOI: 10.1371/journal.pone.0218720

[9] Tan B, Tan N, Koh V, Poh L, Medalia A. Integrative Neuro-Social Cognitive Strategy Programme for Instilling Recovery (INSPIRE): A Community-Based Cognitive Remediation Trial—Study Protocol. Durham, North Carolina, USA: Research Square; 2024. DOI: 10.21203/rs.3.rs-4445167/v1

[10] Nuechterlein KH, McEwen S, Ventura J, Subotnik KL, Turner LR, Boucher M, et al. Aerobic exercise enhances cognitive training effects in first-episode schizophrenia: Randomized clinical trial demonstrates cognitive and functional gains. Psychological Medicine. 2022;**53**(10):4751-4761. DOI: 10.1017/s0033291722001696

[11] Lepage M, Bodnar M, Bowie C. Neurocognition: Clinical

and functional outcomes in schizophrenia. The Canadian Journal of Psychiatry. 2014;**59**(1):5-12. DOI: 10.1177/070674371405900103

[12] Tripathi A, Kar S, Shukla R. Cognitive deficits in schizophrenia: understanding the biological correlates and remediation strategies. Clinical Psychopharmacology and Neuroscience. 2018;**16**(1):7-17. DOI: 10.9758/cpn.2018.16.1.7

[13] Ferrarelli F, Riedner BA, Peterson MJ, Tononi G. Altered prefrontal activity and connectivity predict different cognitive deficits in schizophrenia. Human Brain Mapping. 2015;**36**(11):4539-4552. DOI: 10.1002/hbm.22935

[14] Saxena A, Patel D, Ayesha IE, Monson NR, Klair N, Patel U, et al. Metabolic syndrome causing cognitive impairment in patients with schizophrenia: A systematic review. Cureus. 2023;**15**(10):e47587. DOI: 10.7759/cureus.47587

[15] Zanelli J, Reichenberg A, Sandin S, Morgan C, Dazzan P, Pilecka I, et al. Dynamic and static cognitive deficits in schizophrenia and bipolar disorder after the first episode. Schizophrenia Bulletin. 2022;**48**(3):590-598. DOI: 10.1093/schbul/sbab150

[16] Burton C, Harvey P, Patterson T, Twamley E. Neurocognitive insight and objective cognitive functioning in schizophrenia. Schizophrenia Research. 2016;**171**(1-3):131-136. DOI: 10.1016/j.schres.2016.01.021

[17] Hart X, Mitsukura Y, Bies R, Uchida H. Unraveling the influence of age, IQ, education, and negative symptoms on neurocognitive performance in schizophrenia: A conditional inference tree analysis. Pharmacopsychiatry. 2024;**57**(02):53-60. DOI: 10.1055/a-2258-0379

[18] Priyamvada R, Ranjan R, Jha G. Correlation of neurocognitive deficits with positive and negative symptoms in schizophrenia. Industrial Psychiatry Journal. 2021;**30**(2):249-254. DOI: 10.4103/ipj.ipj_44_20

[19] Minor K, Lysaker P. Necessary, but not sufficient: Links between neurocognition, social cognition, and metacognition in schizophrenia are moderated by disorganized symptoms. Schizophrenia Research. 2014;**159**(1):198-204. DOI: 10.1016/j.schres.2014.08.005

[20] Lam BYH, Raine A, Lee TMC. The relationship between neurocognition and symptomatology in people with schizophrenia: Social cognition as the mediator. BMC Psychiatry. 2014;**14**:138. DOI: 10.1186/1471-244x-14-138

[21] Hemager N, Plessen KJ, Thorup A, Christiani C, Ellersgaard D, Spang KS, et al. Assessment of neurocognitive functions in 7-year-old children at familial high risk for schizophrenia or bipolar disorder: The Danish High Risk and Resilience Study VIA 7. JAMA Psychiatry. 2018;**75**(8):844-852. DOI: 10.1001/jamapsychiatry.2018.1415

[22] Okasha TA, Hussein H, Shorub E, et al. Cognitive dysfunction among inpatients and outpatients with schizophrenia: Relationship to positive and negative symptoms. Middle East Current Psychiatry. 2020;**27**:58. DOI: 10.1186/s43045-020-00062-9

[23] Haugen I, Stubberud J, Ueland T, Haug E, Glenne ØM. Executive dysfunction in schizophrenia: Predictors of the discrepancy between subjective and objective measures. Schizophrenia Research: Cognition. 2021;**26**:100201. DOI: 10.1016/j.scog.2021.100201

[24] Juola P, Salo H, Murray G, Ahmed A, Veijola J, Isohanni M, et al. Neurocognition as a predictor of outcome in schizophrenia in the northern finland birth cohort 1966. Schizophrenia Research: Cognition. 2015;**2**(3):113-119. DOI: 10.1016/j.scog.2015.07.001

[25] Knudsen C, Hemager N, Greve A, Lambek R, Andreassen A, Veddum L, et al. Neurocognitive development in children at familial high risk of schizophrenia or bipolar disorder. JAMA Psychiatry. 2022;**79**(6):589. DOI: 10.1001/jamapsychiatry.2022.0465

[26] Lesh T, Niendam T, Minzenberg M, Carter C. Cognitive control deficits in schizophrenia: Mechanisms and meaning. Neuropsychopharmacology. 2010;**36**(1):316-338. DOI: 10.1038/npp.2010.156

[27] Peng P, Wang D, Wang Q, Zhou Y, Hao Y, Chen S, et al. Alexithymia in chinese patients with chronic schizophrenia: Prevalence, clinical correlates, and relationship with neurocognition and empathy. Asia-Pacific. Psychiatry. 2023;**15**(4):e12547. DOI: 10.1111/appy.12547

[28] Yu Y, Yun Z, Si Y, Ren Q, Ren W, Jing C, et al. Estimation of the cool executive function using frontal electroencephalogram signals in first-episode schizophrenia patients. Biomedical Engineering Online. 2016;**15**(1):131. DOI: 10.1186/s12938-016-0282-y

[29] Kern R, Gold J, Dickinson D, Green M, Nuechterlein K, Baade L, et al. The mccb impairment profile for schizophrenia outpatients: Results from the matrics psychometric and standardization study. Schizophrenia Research. 2011;**126**(1-3):124-131. DOI: 10.1016/j.schres.2010.11.008

[30] Fett A, Viechtbauer W, Domínguez M, Penn D, Os J, Krabbendam L. The relationship between neurocognition and social cognition with functional outcomes in schizophrenia: A meta-analysis. Neuroscience and Biobehavioral Reviews. 2011;**35**(3):573-588. DOI: 10.1016/j.neubiorev.2010.07.001

[31] Abi-Dargham A, Rodenhiser J, Printz D, Zea-Ponce Y, Gil R, Kegeles L, et al. Increased baseline occupancy of D2 receptors by dopamine in schizophrenia. Proceedings of the National Academy of Sciences of the United States of America. 2000;**97**(14):8104-8109. DOI: 10.1073/pnas.97.14.8104

[32] McCutcheon R, Marques T, Howes O. Schizophrenia—An overview. JAMA Psychiatry. 2020;**77**(2):201. DOI: 10.1001/jamapsychiatry.2019.3360

[33] Smucny J, Dienel SJ, Lewis DA, et al. Mechanisms underlying dorsolateral prefrontal cortex contributions to cognitive dysfunction in schizophrenia. Neuropsychopharmacology. 2022;**47**:292-308. DOI: 10.1038/s41386-021-01089-0

[34] Rao N, Northoff G, Tagore A, Rusjan P, Kenk M, Wilson A, et al. Impaired prefrontal cortical dopamine release in schizophrenia during a cognitive task: A [11C]FLB 457 positron emission tomography study. Schizophrenia Bulletin. 2019;**45**(3):670-679. DOI: 10.1093/schbul/sby076

[35] Zhang Q. Stress, dopamine and the development of schizophrenia. Lecture Notes in Education Psychology and Public Media. 2024;**33**(1):215-220. DOI: 10.54254/2753-7048/33/20231749

[36] Purves-Tyson T, Owens SJ, Rothmond DA, Halliday GM, Double KL, Stevens J, et al. Putative presynaptic dopamine dysregulation in

schizophrenia is supported by molecular evidence from post-mortem human midbrain. Translational Psychiatry. 2017;7(1):e1003. DOI: 10.1038/tp.2016.257

[37] Al-Asmary SM, Kadasah S, Arfin M, Tariq M, Alasmari A. Genetic association of catechol-O-methyltransferase Val(158)Met polymorphism in Saudi schizophrenia patients. Genetics and Molecular Research. 2014;**13**(2):3079-3088. DOI: 10.4238/2014.April.17.4

[38] Dahoun T, Trossbach SV, Brandon NJ, Korth C, Howes O. The impact of disrupted-in-schizophrenia 1 (DISC1) on the dopaminergic system: A systematic review. Translational Psychiatry. 2017;7(1):e1015. DOI: 10.1038/tp.2016.282

[39] Heinz A, Schlagenhauf F. Dopaminergic dysfunction in schizophrenia: Salience attribution revisited. Schizophrenia Bulletin. 2010;**36**(3):472-485. DOI: 10.1093/schbul/sbq031

[40] Stilo SA, Murray RM. Non-genetic factors in schizophrenia. Current Psychiatry Reports. 2019;**21**(10):109. DOI: 10.1007/s11920-019-1091-3

[41] Stone J, Morrison P, Pilowsky LS. Glutamate and dopamine dysregulation in schizophrenia: A synthesis and selective review. Journal of Psychopharmacology. 2006;**21**(4):440-452. DOI: 10.1177/0269881106073126

[42] Ferdinand J, Peters KZ, Yavas E, Young AMJ. Modulation of stimulated dopamine release in rat nucleus accumbens shell by GABA in vitro: Effect of sub-chronic phencyclidine pretreatment. Journal of Neuroscience Research. 2021;**99**(7):1885-1901. DOI: 10.1002/jnr.24843

[43] Noda Y, Barr MS, Zomorrodi R, Cash R, Rajji TK, Farzan F, et al. Reduced short-latency afferent inhibition in prefrontal but not motor cortex and its association with executive function in schizophrenia: A combined TMS-EEG study. Schizophrenia Bulletin. 2017;**44**(1):193-202. DOI: 10.1093/schbul/sbx041

[44] Carruthers SP, Gurvich CT, Rossell SL. The muscarinic system, cognition and schizophrenia. Neuroscience and Biobehavioral Reviews. 2015;**55**:393-402. DOI: 10.1016/j.neubiorev.2015.05.008

[45] Bansal V, Chatterjee I. Role of neurotransmitters in schizophrenia: A comprehensive study. Kuwait Journal of Science. 2021;**48**(2):1-27. DOI: 10.48129/kjs.v48i2.9264

[46] Wyss C, Hitz K, Hengartner MP, Theodoridou A, Obermann C, Uhl I, et al. The loudness dependence of auditory evoked potentials (LDAEP) as an indicator of serotonergic dysfunction in patients with predominant schizophrenic negative symptoms. PLoS One. 2013;**8**(7):e68650. DOI: 10.1371/journal.pone.0068650

[47] Moghaddam B, Javitt DC. From revolution to evolution: The glutamate hypothesis of schizophrenia and its implication for treatment. Neuropsychopharmacology. 2011;**37**(1):4-15. DOI: 10.1038/npp.2011.181

[48] Coyle JT, Basu AC, Benneyworth MA, Balu DT, Konopaske G. Glutamatergic synaptic dysregulation in schizophrenia: Therapeutic implications. Handbook of Experimental Pharmacology. 2012;(213):267-295. DOI: 10.1007/978-3-642-25758-2_10

[49] Liu Y, Chen J, Huang L, Yan S, Bian Q, Yang F. Relationships among

retinal nerve fiber layer thickness, vascular endothelial growth factor, and cognitive impairment in patients with schizophrenia. Neuropsychiatric Disease and Treatment. 2021;**17**:3597-3606. DOI: 10.2147/ndt.s336077

[50] Pillai A, Howell KR, Ahmed AO, Weinberg D, Allen KM, Bruggemann J, et al. Association of serum VEGF levels with prefrontal cortex volume in schizophrenia. Molecular Psychiatry. 2015;**21**(5):686-692. DOI: 10.1038/mp.2015.96

[51] Howell KR, Kutiyanawalla A, Pillai A. Long-term continuous corticosterone treatment decreases VEGF receptor-2 expression in frontal cortex. PLoS One. 2011;**6**(5):e20198. DOI: 10.1371/journal.pone.0020198

[52] Howell KR, Pillai A. Effects of prenatal hypoxia on schizophrenia-related phenotypes in heterozygous reeler mice: A gene × environment interaction study. European Neuropsychopharmacology. 2014;**24**(8):1324-1336. DOI: 10.1016/j.euroneuro.2014.05.011

[53] Lee BH, Hong JP, Hwang J, Ham BJ, Lee J, Kim WJ, et al. Alterations in plasma vascular endothelial growth factor levels in patients with schizophrenia before and after treatment. Psychiatry Research. 2015;**228**(1):95-99. DOI: 10.1016/j.psychres.2015.04.020

[54] Norton N, Moskvina V, Morris DW, Bray NJ, Zammit S, Williams N, et al. Evidence that interaction between neuregulin 1 and its receptor ErbB4 increases susceptibility to schizophrenia. American Journal of Medical Genetics. Part B, Neuropsychiatric Genetics. 2005;**141B**(1):96-101. DOI: 10.1002/ajmg.b.30236

[55] Yang H, Wen P, Xiao W, Yang M, Xu J, Li J, et al. Antipsychotic drugs increase neuregulin1β1 serum levels in first-episode drug-naïve patients and chronic schizophrenia with suggestions for improving the treatment of psychotic symptoms. BMC Psychiatry. 2022;**22**(1):1-11. DOI: 10.1186/s12888-022-03856-9

[56] Pitcher G, Kalia LV, Ng D, Goodfellow NM, Yee KT, Lambe EK, et al. Schizophrenia susceptibility pathway neuregulin 1–ErbB4 suppresses Src upregulation of NMDA receptors. Nature Medicine. 2011;**17**(4):470-478. DOI: 10.1038/nm.2315

[57] Geddes AE, Huang X, Newell KA. Reciprocal signalling between NR2 subunits of the NMDA receptor and neuregulin1 and their role in schizophrenia. Progress in Neuro-Psychopharmacology & Biological Psychiatry. 2011;**35**(4):896-904. DOI: 10.1016/j.pnpbp.2011.02.017

[58] Du N, Meng X, Li J, Shi L, Chen L, Yao L, et al. Decline in Working Memory in Stable Schizophrenia May be Related to Attentional Impairment: Mediating Effects of Negative Symptoms. Durham, North Carolina, USA: Research Square; 2023. DOI: 10.21203/rs.3.rs-3224248/v1

[59] Madeira N, Caldeira S, Bajouco M, Pereira A, Martins MJ, Macedo A. Social cognition, negative symptoms and psychosocial functioning in schizophrenia. International Journal of Clinical Neurosciences and Mental Health. 2016;**3**:1. DOI: 10.21035/ijcnmh.2016.3.1

[60] Andrzejewska M, Wójciak P, Domowicz K, Rybakowski J. Emotion recognition and theory of mind in chronic schizophrenia: Association with negative symptoms. Archives of Psychiatry and Psychotherapy. 2017;**19**(4):7-12. DOI: 10.12740/app/79878

[61] Krishnadas R, Ramanathan S, Wong E, Nayak AK, Moore BP. Residual negative symptoms differentiate cognitive performance in clinically stable patients with schizophrenia and bipolar disorder. Schizophrenia Research and Treatment. 2014;**2014**:1-6. DOI: 10.1155/2014/785310

[62] Bliksted V, Videbech P, Fagerlund B, Frith CD. The effect of positive symptoms on social cognition in first-episode schizophrenia is modified by the presence of negative symptoms. Neuropsychology. 2017;**31**(2):209-219. DOI: 10.1037/neu0000309

[63] Montvidas J, Adomaitienė V, Leskauskas D, Dollfus S. Correlation of health-related quality of life with negative symptoms assessed with the self-evaluation of negative symptoms scale (SNS) and cognitive deficits in schizophrenia: A cross-sectional study in routine psychiatric care. Journal of Clinical Medicine. 2023;**12**(3):901. DOI: 10.3390/jcm12030901

[64] Charernboon T. Interplay among positive and negative symptoms, neurocognition, social cognition, and functioning in clinically stable patients with schizophrenia: A network analysis. F1000Research. 2022;**10**:1258. DOI: 10.12688/f1000research.74385.2

[65] Bora E, Akdede BB, Alptekın K. Neurocognitive impairment in deficit and non-deficit schizophrenia: A meta-analysis. Psychological Medicine. 2017;**47**(14):2401-2413. DOI: 10.1017/s0033291717000952

[66] Mete L, Sarikaya O, Erol A. The relationship of deficit syndrome with clinical symptoms, summer births and heritability in patients with schizophrenia. Turkish Journal of Psychiatry. 2015;**26**(4):229-235. DOI: 10.5080/u11182

[67] Wang P, Cai J, Ni J, Zhang J, Tang W, Zhang C. The NCAN gene: Schizophrenia susceptibility and cognitive dysfunction. Neuropsychiatric Disease and Treatment. 2016;**12**:2875-2883. DOI: 10.2147/ndt.s118160

[68] Sheffield JM, Karcher NR, Deanna M. Cognitive deficits in psychotic disorders: A lifespan perspective. Neuropsychology Review. 2018;**28**(4):509-533. DOI: 10.1007/s11065-018-9388-2

[69] Green MF, Horan WP, Lee J. Nonsocial and social cognition in schizophrenia: Current evidence and future directions. World Psychiatry. 2019;**18**(2):146-161. DOI: 10.1002/wps.20624

[70] Wu Q, Wang X, Wang Y, Long Y, Zhao J, Wu R. Developments in biological mechanisms and treatments for negative symptoms and cognitive dysfunction of schizophrenia. Neuroscience Bulletin. 2021;**37**(11):1609-1624. DOI: 10.1007/s12264-021-00740-6

[71] Barlati S, Deste G, Gregorelli M, Vita A. Autistic traits in a sample of adult patients with schizophrenia: Prevalence and correlates. Psychological Medicine. 2018;**49**(1):140-148. DOI: 10.1017/s0033291718000600

Section 2

Scientific Foundations of Psychosis

Chapter 3

Neural Substrates of Psychosis and Cognitive Impairment in Mouse Models of Schizophrenia

Maria Victoria Puig, Thomas Gener, Cristina López-Cabezón and Sara Hidalgo-Nieves

Abstract

Schizophrenia is a multifaceted psychiatric disorder characterized by positive, negative, and cognitive symptoms. While its cellular mechanisms remain elusive, the prefrontal cortex (PFC) and hippocampus (HPC) are central to the disorder's pathophysiology, with patients showing structural and functional anomalies in these regions. We examined aberrant neural activity within prefrontal-hippocampal circuits in mice treated with phencyclidine (PCP), a psychostimulant that produces schizophrenia symptoms in humans and rodents. Acute PCP administration induced psychosis that correlated with prefrontal hypersynchronization, hippocampal desynchronization, and disrupted circuit connectivity. The atypical antipsychotic risperidone alleviated cortical disturbances with minimal impact on the HPC, whereas the classical neuroleptic haloperidol exacerbated circuit disruptions, revealing distinct effects of atypical and classical APDs on prefrontal-hippocampal dynamics. Notably, serotonin 5-HT_{2A}R antagonism and 5-HT_{1A}R agonism outperformed risperidone in restoring prefrontal-hippocampal dynamics. Subchronic PCP treatment produced enduring cognitive impairments, including deficits in short- and long-term memory, auditory processing and attention, which were accompanied by increased prefrontal and reduced hippocampal neural synchronization. Chronic risperidone improved impaired memory and auditory processing, but not auditory attention, while mitigating hippocampal disturbances, providing a neural framework for its cognitive benefits in schizophrenia. These findings suggest that cortical hypersynchronization contributes to positive symptoms, whereas hippocampal desynchronization and disrupted connectivity underlie cognitive deficits in schizophrenia.

Keywords: NMDAR hypofunction, serotonin receptors, antipsychotic drug, neural synchrony, oscillopathy, theta and gamma oscillations, phase coherence, phase-amplitude coupling, spike-LFP coherence, recognition memory, auditory processing, *in vivo* electrophysiology

1. Introduction

Schizophrenia is a debilitating disorder associated with chronic disability and premature mortality. A major challenge for individuals with schizophrenia is its complex symptomatology, which is inadequately addressed by current pharmacological treatments. Patients are typically diagnosed in adolescence or early adulthood, following the onset of psychosis (positive symptoms). However, by this time, many of them already exhibit a history of emotional and cognitive impairments (negative and cognitive symptoms, respectively). This constellation of clinical manifestations complicates treatment, particularly given that most antipsychotic drugs effectively reduce positive symptoms but have little or no impact on other impairments. In fact, some antipsychotics may even exacerbate emotional and cognitive distress. Decades of research have provided invaluable insights into the anatomical and functional brain alterations that are likely to contribute to the disease. Among these, the prefrontal cortex (PFC), located in the brain's frontal regions, has been widely recognized for its fundamental role. Post-mortem studies of brains from individuals with schizophrenia have revealed reductions in cortical thickness and deficits in neural circuitry, particularly in inhibitory neurons [1, 2]. These abnormalities, however, cannot fully explain the diverse clinical features of the illness, limiting drug discovery efforts. Therefore, there is an urgent need to develop novel research strategies.

Our group has adopted several research approaches to overcome some of these limitations: (1) we focus on brain circuits rather than isolated brain regions; (2) we investigate aberrant neural dynamics during a variety of abnormal behaviors relevant to schizophrenia within the same individual; and (3) we leverage the effects of different antipsychotic medications to identify neural dynamics susceptible to becoming useful biomarkers for diagnosis and treatment. Through these studies, we also aim to provide new insights into the strengths and limitations of various types of antipsychotic drugs, including classical neuroleptics and atypical antipsychotics. To achieve this efficiently, we utilize preclinical models of schizophrenia, which allow for the implantation of recording electrodes in specific brain regions of interest enabling thorough monitoring of changes in neural dynamics as animals exhibit behaviors relevant to the disorder.

Our research has focused on a brain circuit connecting the PFC with the hippocampus (HPC), the brain's central memory hub. Given the PFC's critical role in orchestrating executive functions [3], the prefrontal-hippocampal circuit is particularly relevant to both the positive and cognitive symptoms of schizophrenia. Disruption of neural communication between these regions may represent a core feature not only of schizophrenia but also other neuropsychiatric disorders. Local neural activities are also disrupted in schizophrenia patients. More specifically, neural networks oscillating at gamma frequencies are altered in several cortical regions. These oscillations are prominent during routine cognitive processes such as sensory perception and attention, and their disruption has been associated with both hallucinations and cognitive deficits in patients [4–8]. However, a limitation of these studies is that neural dynamics were investigated using EEG, which average neural signals across extensive brain areas, potentially masking localized circuit-level effects. In contrast, invasive experimentation in rodent models allows for more precise investigation of specific brain regions and the effects of targeted genetic and cellular manipulations. Preclinical studies have highlighted the potential involvement of prefrontal-hippocampal circuits in the pathophysiology of schizophrenia and other psychiatric disorders [9, 10].

We investigated two critical subregions within prefrontal and hippocampal microcircuits relevant to psychosis and cognitive deficits: the prelimbic medial prefrontal cortex (mPFC) and the CA1 region of the dorsal hippocampus (dHPC). In rodents, the mPFC sends direct afferent inputs to the CA1 area, while the reverse pathway involves the nucleus reuniens of the thalamus [10]. Remarkably, this circuit exhibits strong intrinsic neural synchronization within the theta and gamma frequency ranges that can be used to investigate pathophysiological mechanisms and the effects of medication [11–15]. We employed a pharmacological model of schizophrenia based on the hypofunction of N-methyl-D-aspartate glutamate receptors (NMDARs), a cellular mechanism considered a critical element in the pathophysiology of the disorder. NMDAR antagonists are widely used to model schizophrenia in both humans and animal studies as they effectively replicate many of the disorder's core positive, negative, and cognitive symptoms. For instance, acute administration of the NMDAR antagonist ketamine induces transient psychotic symptoms in healthy individuals and worsens pre-existing symptoms in schizophrenia patients [16, 17]. Similarly, in rodents, acute NMDAR antagonism with ketamine or phencyclidine (PCP, also known as angel dust) produces abnormal behaviors resembling the positive symptoms of schizophrenia [18, 19]. Chronic administration of NMDAR blockers results in sustained cognitive deficits, including impairments in memory and sensory processing -cognitive domains similarly affected in schizophrenia patients [19, 20]. We leveraged the unique features of the PCP pharmacological model to dissect the contributions of prefrontal-hippocampal circuits to psychosis and cognitive impairments in mice. We aimed to provide new insights into the distinct roles of these circuits in schizophrenia symptoms, offering a framework for evaluating novel therapeutic strategies.

2. Neural substrates of psychosis in mice

2.1 The phencyclidine model of psychosis

Acute administration of PCP to rodents induces robust psychotomimetic effects. In our studies, we administered a single subcutaneous (s.c.) injection of 10 mg/kg PCP to freely moving mice. This model of psychosis is highly reliable, eliciting psychotic-like behaviors in 100% of the animals within 10–15 minutes, and has been used for decades to investigate the effects of antipsychotic drugs (APDs) [19, 20]. To validate this model under our experimental conditions, which included electrophysiological recordings, mice were implanted with two pairs of tungsten electrodes (called stereotrodes) in the prelimbic PFC (mPFC) and the CA1 region of the HPC (dHPC). During the experiments, the electrodes were connected to a data acquisition system via a thin, flexible cable (**Figure 1**).

In separate experiments conducted 1 week apart, we administered either saline (as a control) or the APD risperidone (0.5 mg/kg, intraperitoneally [i.p.]) 15 minutes after PCP injection and recorded neural activities for 1 hour. As anticipated, PCP administration increased locomotor activity (distance traveled) and stereotypic behaviors (repetitive movements), both of which were significantly attenuated by risperidone. Conversely, PCP-induced ataxia (movement discoordination) was initially exacerbated by risperidone before eventually aligning with the effects of PCP. These behavioral alterations corresponded with mild reductions in accelerometer data, collected via sensors integrated into the headstages of the electrophysiological system, that were exacerbated by risperidone. Collectively, these findings validate the PCP model of psychosis under our experimental conditions and highlight its utility in investigating the neural dynamics underlying psychotic behaviors and the therapeutic effects of APDs.

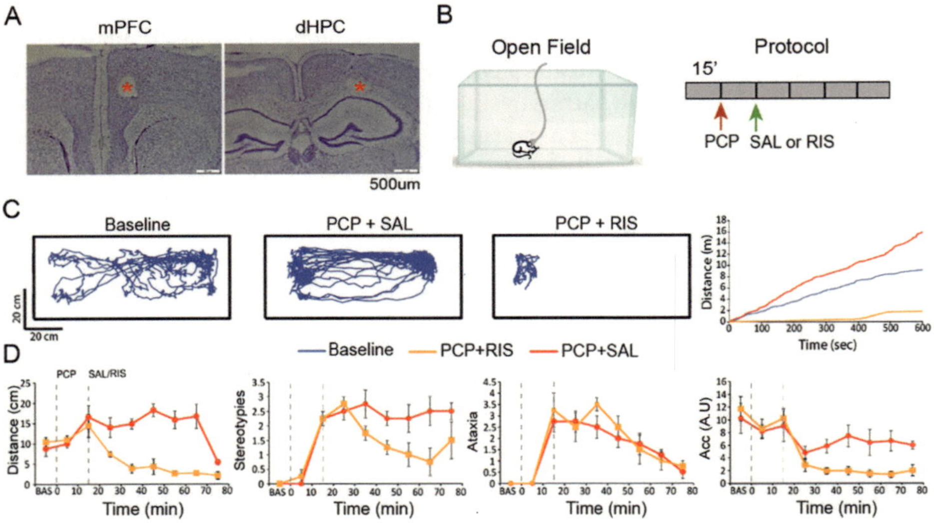

Figure 1.
Acute PCP induced psychosis-like behaviors in mice that were reduced by the APD risperidone. (A) Mice were implanted with recording electrodes in the prelimbic mPFC and the CA1 area of the dHPC. Correct electrode placement was confirmed via cresyl violet staining of brain slices. In this example, the electrode tip locations are marked with asterisks. (B) During the experimental sessions, mice were connected to an electrophysiology system via a flexible cable. PCP (10 mg/kg, s.c.) was administered while the mice explored an open field. Saline (SAL) or risperidone (RIS, 0.5 mg/kg, i.p.) were injected 15 minutes after PCP in separate sessions. Behavioral activity was monitored for 1 hour following the administration of saline or risperidone. (C) Representative 10-min locomotion traces are shown for baseline, PCP + SAL, and PCP + RIS sessions. During PCP + SAL sessions, mice exhibited marked hyperlocomotion, as indicated by the cumulative distance traveled (right panel). This hyperactivity was significantly attenuated in PCP + RIS sessions. (D) PCP induced hyperlocomotion and stereotypies for at least 1 hour, that were mitigated by risperidone. Ataxia also increased but was not rescued by the APD. Accelerometer readings are also shown. Modified from [13].

2.2 Natural coordination of the mPFC and the dHPC *in vivo*

The mPFC and the dHPC exhibit highly coordinated neural activity *in vivo*, with consistent patterns observed across animals. This coordination is revealed by combining electrophysiological recordings with advanced mathematical methods that assess changes in neural synchronization, both within local brain areas and across circuit-level interactions (**Table 1**). The *power* of neural oscillations, which reflects the amplitude of oscillatory waves, is represented by spectrograms, color-maps that display frequency power (typically ranging from 0.1 to 200 Hz or more) over time (measured in seconds or minutes) (**Figure 2**). Spectrograms typically show red and yellow colors at low frequencies (delta, theta, and alpha bands), indicating large amplitudes, while higher frequencies (low, high gamma, and high frequency bands) appear in blue, reflecting smaller amplitudes. This pattern follows the 1/f power law [21]. Within this natural gradient of power, several distinct oscillatory bands can be readily identified. During normal wakefulness, neural oscillations in the HPC typically exhibit larger amplitudes than those in the PFC, particularly below 100 Hz. Notably, a well-defined theta band (7–9 Hz) in the HPC strongly correlates with animal locomotion (**Table 2**) [26].

Another important measure of neural synchronization is cross-frequency *phase-amplitude coupling* (PAC). PAC reflects the modulation of fast oscillations (50–250 Hz) by the phase of slower oscillations (2–16 Hz) [22], and can be

Measure (abbreviation)	Description	Domain	Ref.	Diagram
Power spectral density (PSD)	Quantifies the distribution of signal power across frequencies	Local	[21]	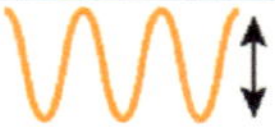
Phase-amplitude coupling (PAC)	Measures how the phase of one frequency modulates the amplitude of another	Local and circuit	[22]	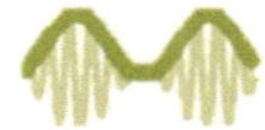
Pairwise phase consistency (PPC)	Evaluates the synchronization between spikes and oscillations	Local	[23]	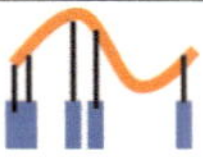
Weighted phase-lag index (wPLI)	Measures strength and consistency of phase relationships between regions	Circuit	[24]	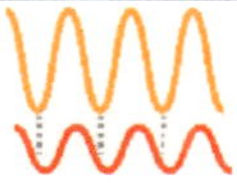
Phase slope index (PSI)	Determines the directionality of information flow between regions	Circuit	[25]	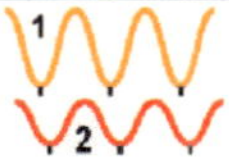

Table 1.
Summary of electrophysiological measures used to assess neural synchronization in local and circuit domains.

assessed both locally within a brain region and across regions (i.e., the amplitude of high-frequency oscillations in one area is modulated by the phase of low-frequency oscillations in another area). Within the HPC, theta-gamma coupling is particularly prominent and sensitive to both pharmacological and environmental manipulations. For instance, it is disrupted by antipsychotic drugs and enhanced by cognitive stimulation [13, 15]. This coupling may play critical roles in memory processes such as encoding, retrieval and consolidation [27–30]. *Spike-local field potential (LFP) coherence* provides another measure of neural coordination by quantifying the synchronization of action potentials with ongoing oscillations. Here, we estimated spike-LFP coherence using the pairwise phase consistency method [23]. Neurons in the dHPC show strong synchronization with ongoing theta, beta, and low gamma oscillations, while in the mPFC many neurons fire action potentials in coordination with delta waves (**Table 2**).

At the circuit level, *phase coherence* measures the synchronization of oscillations within the same frequency band across regions. We used the weighted phase-lag index (wPLI) method, which accounts for the removal of common source zero-lag effects, reducing contamination from signals that may affect multiple regions simultaneously [24]. In healthy mice, coherence between the theta (7–9 Hz) and low gamma (25–40 Hz) bands is consistently detectable. To assess *signal directionality* within the circuit, we used the phase slope index (PSI) method [25], which estimates the consistency (low variance) of the phase lag between two signals within a given frequency band. If there is a consistent phase relationship between the two signals, the variance in phase lag is significantly smaller than that of surrogate data. The sign of the phase relationship indicates which signal leads or lags the other, thus providing a measure of directionality. In our studies, we defined positive slopes as dHPC → mPFC (dark red) and negative slopes as mPFC → dHPC (green) directions of signal flow. In awake, healthy mice, a robust dHPC → mPFC theta band (4–10 Hz) is consistently detected, which appears as a wide dark red band in the directionally color plots.

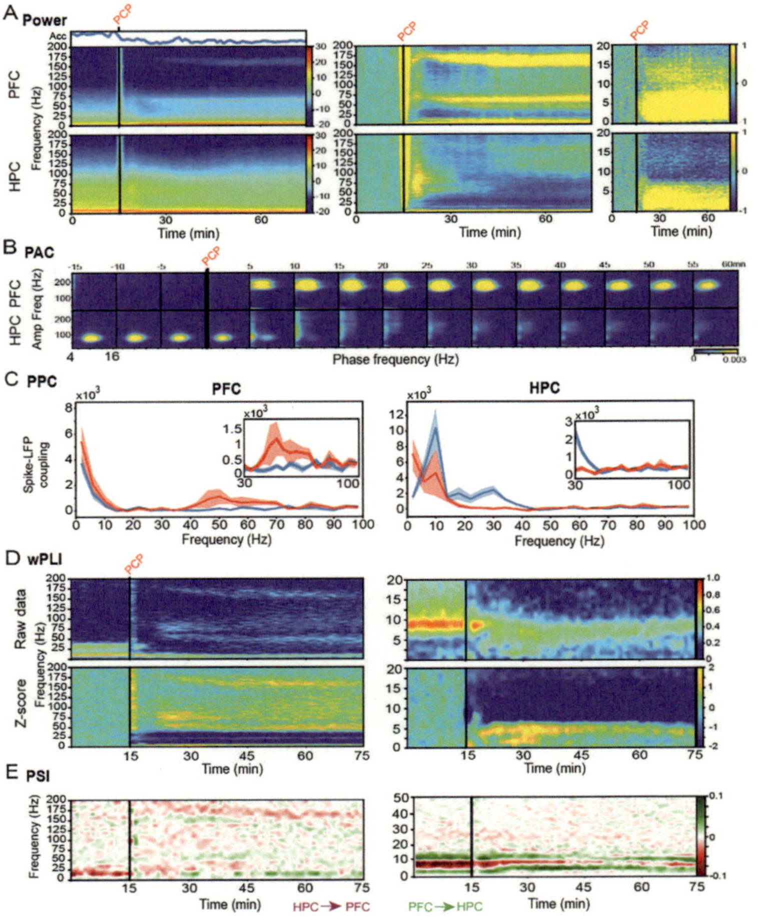

Figure 2.
Acute PCP enhanced prefrontal and disrupted hippocampal neural synchronization, and impaired circuit connectivity. (A) Power spectrograms: Time course of power changes in the mPFC (top) and dHPC (bottom) following PCP administration (10 mg/kg, s.c.). Left panels display raw data alongside the animals' mobility quantified via the accelerometer (Acc). Middle and right panels show z-scores relative to baseline, highlighting distinct activity patterns. (B) Cross-frequency coupling (PAC): time course of local phase-amplitude coupling maps in consecutive 5-minute epochs. The x-axis represents phase frequencies, while the y-axis represents amplitude frequencies. (C) Spike-local field potential coherence (PPC): average spike-LFP coherence during baseline (blue) and the 50–60 minute window following PCP administration (red). Note the varying scales across plots. (D) Phase coherence (wPLI): time course of phase coherence changes (raw data and z-scores), indicating alterations in connectivity strength within the circuit. (E) Signal directionality (PSI): Time course of directional connectivity between mPFC and dHPC. Signals from dHPC → mPFC are shown in dark red, while mPFC → dHPC signals are in green, revealing disruptions in circuit dynamics post-PCP. Modified from [13].

2.3 Prefrontal-hippocampal neural dynamics during psychosis

We investigated the effects of PCP (10 mg/kg, s.c.) administration on neural signals in the mPFC and dHPC, as well as on the synchronization of the circuit. PCP administration led to increased neural synchronization in the mPFC but decreased synchronization in the dHPC, while the overall coordination of the circuit was severely disrupted (**Figure 2**) [13]. In the mPFC, several aberrant oscillatory bands emerged: a theta band (8 Hz), an alpha band (12 Hz), and prominent bands within the high gamma (60 Hz) and high frequency ranges (160 Hz). These bands

Band	Name
>100 Hz	High frequencies
50–100 Hz	High gamma
30–50 Hz	Low gamma
18–30 Hz	Beta
13–18 Hz	Alpha
8–12 Hz	Theta
1–4 Hz	Delta

Table 2.
Standard frequency bands used to define neural oscillations in the mouse healthy brain.

reflected strong hypersynchronization within prefrontal microcircuits induced by PCP. In contrast, in the dHPC, PCP decreased the power of theta (8–12 Hz) and beta (18–25 Hz) oscillations, while briefly increasing high gamma oscillations in a broad frequency band (50–110 Hz). Remarkably, delta oscillations were markedly enhanced in both the mPFC and dHPC, suggesting a significant role of this frequency band in the pathological state of the circuit. The delta activity spanned a wide range from 1 to 8 Hz, including an atypical "fast" delta band with a peak at 6.4 Hz.

Other types of local neural synchronization changed in accordance with the power alterations described above, further highlighting the differential effects of PCP on cortical and hippocampal synchronization (**Figure 2**). Specifically, delta and high-frequency coupling (PAC) emerged in prefrontal regions, while the intrinsic theta-gamma coupling in the dHPC was completely disrupted. Although PCP did not significantly alter the firing rate of individual neurons, it impaired their synchronization with ongoing oscillations. In the mPFC, neuronal spikes became more robustly coordinated with gamma waves, whereas in the dHPC, the intrinsic synchronization to theta, beta, and gamma oscillations weakened. Finally, the coordination of spikes with ongoing delta waves was enhanced in both regions after PCP administration, in line with the observed power changes.

Given the profound disruption of local neural activities in both the mPFC and dHPC induced by PCP, a disturbance in the circuit coordination was anticipated. PCP-induced cortical hypersynchronization enhanced phase coherence in parallel with the mPFC power increases. Interestingly, it also facilitated a flow of information from the dHPC to the mPFC (dHPC → mPFC) at high gamma and higher frequencies. These bottom-up flow of information at very high frequencies is puzzling and current research aims at determining their cellular substrate. In contrast, hippocampal "shut down" dominated the circuit's low-frequency signals (<30 Hz), completely disrupting the intrinsic theta and low gamma communication from the dHPC to the mPFC (dHPC → mPFC). Instead, aberrant phase coherence and mPFC → dHPC flow of information were observed at delta frequencies, with a peak at approximately 5 Hz (**Figure 2**).

Taken together, the emergence of aberrant oscillations, cross-frequency coupling, and spike-oscillation coupling revealed a striking hypersynchronization of cortical microcircuits induced by PCP, while hippocampal microcircuits became desynchronized. Furthermore, the circuit's connectivity at high frequencies increased following cortical hyperexcitation, whereas it was severely disrupted at low frequencies, likely due to hippocampal discoordination. Finally, a novel delta-driven synchronization emerged both locally and the circuit level.

2.4 Effects of antipsychotic drugs on aberrant prefrontal-hippocampal neural dynamics during PCP-induced psychosis

We next investigated whether risperidone and haloperidol (both administered at a dose of 0.5 mg/kg, i.p.) could reverse PCP-induced alterations in prefrontal-hippocampal circuits. These two compounds belong to distinct classes of APDs: risperidone is an atypical APD with a strong affinity for serotonin receptors, while haloperidol is a classical neuroleptic that primarily blocks dopamine D2 receptors. In addition to their antipsychotic effects, atypical APDs are known to alleviate negative and cognitive symptoms in schizophrenia patients, whereas classical neuroleptics can have detrimental effects on these symptoms. Thus, it was crucial to determine whether and how these two classes of antipsychotic drugs influence a brain circuit central to the negative and cognitive symptoms of schizophrenia.

Our findings revealed that risperidone (as well as clozapine, another atypical APD; see [13]) effectively mitigated PCP-induced hypersynchronization in the mPFC (**Figure 3**). It reduced the power and frequency of aberrant delta, theta, high gamma and high-frequency bands, as well as the associated delta-high frequency cross-frequency coupling. Although these abnormal bands were not fully eliminated, the observed reductions in power and frequency suggested that full normalization might have required several hours. In contrast, haloperidol exacerbated abnormal gamma oscillations in the dHPC following PCP administration. Neither drug succeeded in restoring intrinsic neural synchronization in the dHPC, including theta oscillations and theta-gamma coupling. Consistently, risperidone—but not haloperidol—attenuated PCP-enhanced delta and gamma spike-LFP coupling in the mPFC. However, neither drug was able to normalize hippocampal spike-LFP coupling at middle frequencies.

At the circuit level, risperidone decreased the strength and frequency of the aberrant phase coherence and signal directionality in the high gamma and high-frequency ranges, mirroring the observed power changes (**Figure 4**). Notably, clozapine demonstrated superior efficacy than risperidone in restoring mPFC-dHPC connectivity [13]. Haloperidol not only failed to correct the increased circuit connectivity induced by PCP but indeed exacerbated mPFC → dHPC delta signals relative to the saline controls. None of the APDs successfully restored the intrinsic theta-beta coherence characteristic of the circuit under normal conditions.

Overall, these experiments highlight profound differences in how the two families of APDs (atypical vs. classical) affect prefrontal-hippocampal neural dynamics *in vivo* during psychosis. The results suggest that risperidone primarily exerts cortical effects, with only marginal influence on the dHPC, whereas haloperidol appears to have a detrimental effect on the entire circuit. These findings align with the clinical outcomes of both medications. We hypothesized that the affinity of atypical ADPs for serotonin receptors may have played a key role in these observed differences. To explore this further, we investigated how serotonin receptors modulate the prefrontal-hippocampal circuit during PCP-induced psychosis in freely moving mice.

2.5 Effects of serotonin receptors on aberrant prefrontal-hippocampal neural dynamics during psychosis

Serotonin 1A and 2A receptors (5-HT_{1A}Rs and 5-HT_{2A}Rs, respectively) are major targets of antipsychotic medication. Specifically, atypical APDs such as risperidone and clozapine directly block 5-HT_{2A}Rs and indirectly activate 5-HT_{1A}Rs [31, 32].

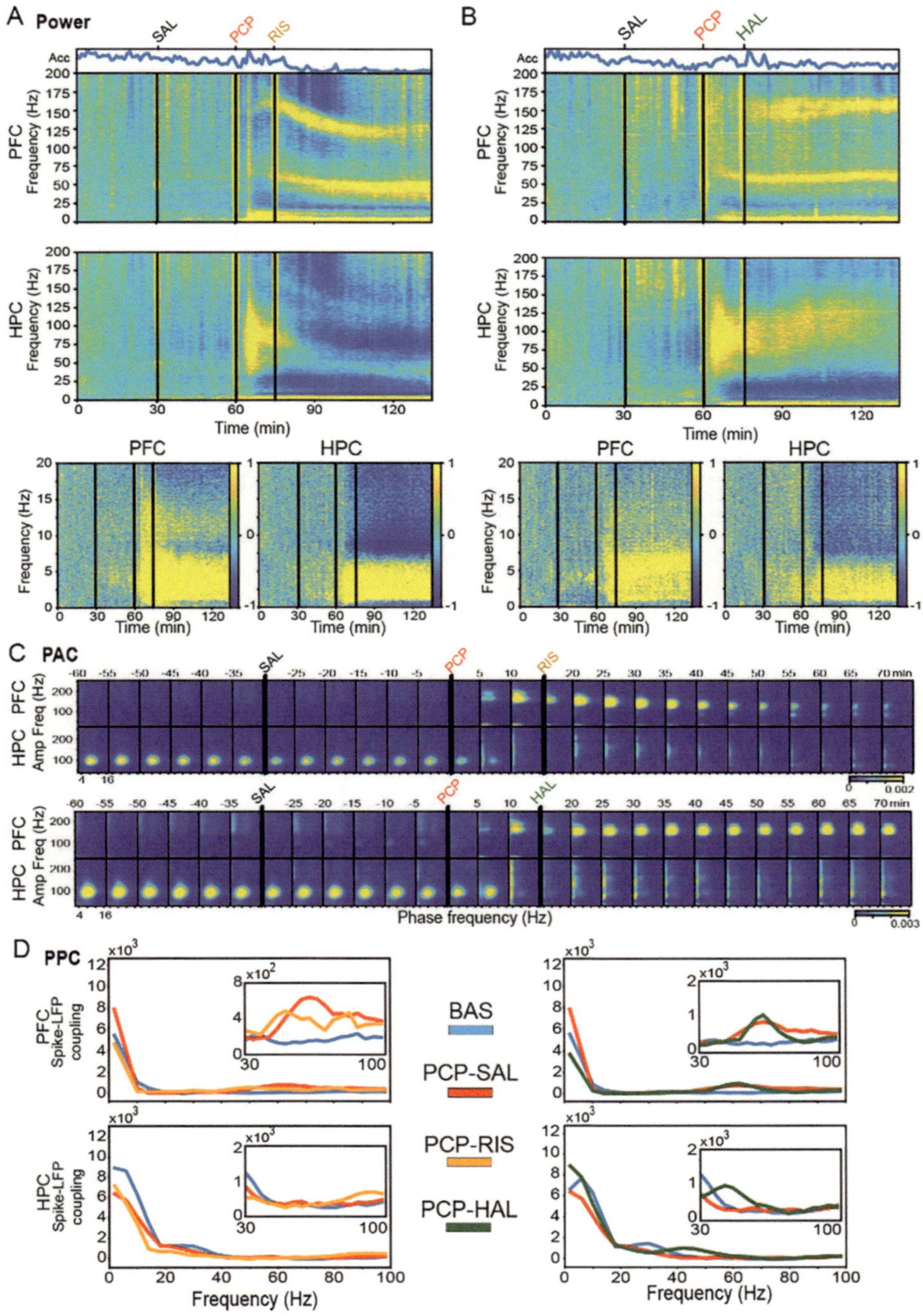

Figure 3.
Risperidone, but not haloperidol, attenuated prefrontal hypersynchronization during PCP-induced psychosis. (A) Risperidone significantly reduced PCP-induced aberrant power in the delta, theta, alpha, and high-frequency bands in the mPFC but did not alleviate hippocampal inhibition. Z-scores relative to baseline are shown. (B) Haloperidol failed to counteract the PCP-induced power alterations and exacerbated hippocampal high gamma oscillations compared to controls. (C) Risperidone mitigated abnormal delta-high frequency coupling in the mPFC, aligning with the observed reductions in power. In contrast, haloperidol worsened this aberrant coupling, highlighting its limited efficacy in addressing these disturbances. Neither drug restored intrinsic theta-gamma coupling in the dHPC. (D) Risperidone attenuated aberrant delta and gamma (inset) spike-LFP coupling in the mPFC, while neither drug rescued hippocampal spike-oscillation coupling at middle frequencies. Modified from [13].

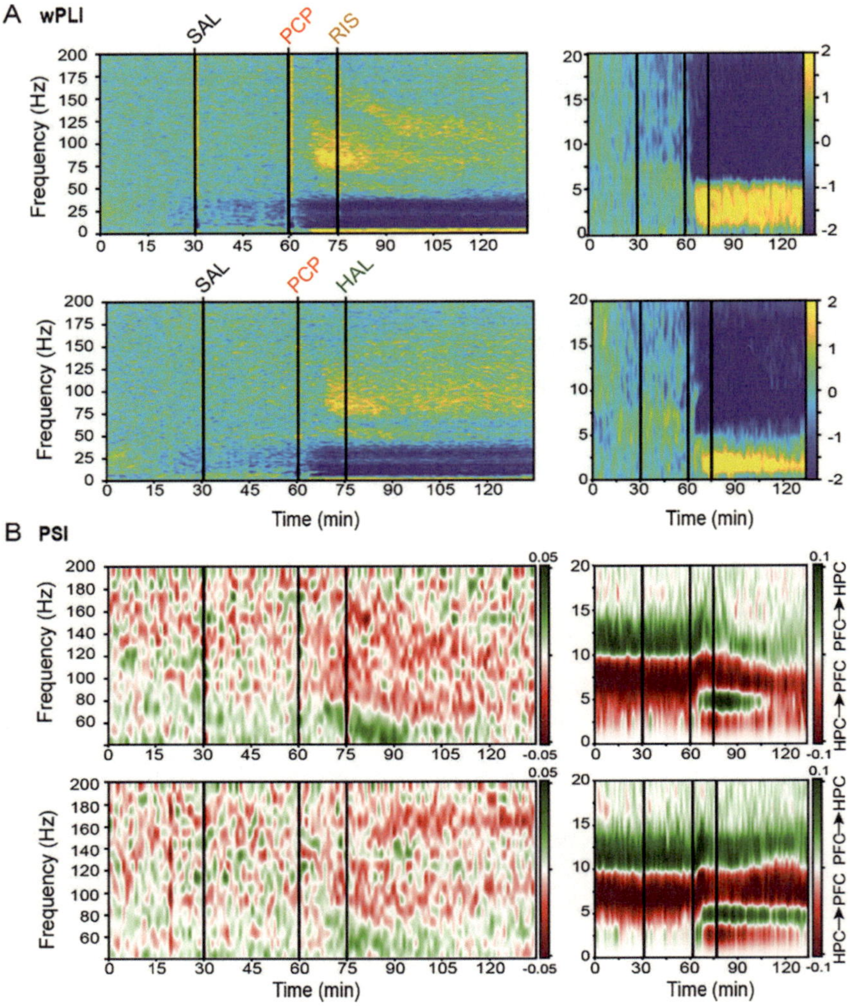

Figure 4.
Risperidone, but not haloperidol, attenuated increased mPFC-dHPC connectivity during PCP-induced psychosis. (A) Risperidone reduced the strength and frequency of aberrant phase coherence in the high gamma and high-frequency ranges relative to baseline but failed to restore synchrony at medium frequencies, which remained markedly suppressed. Elevated delta coherence also persisted. Z-scores relative to baseline are shown. (B) Risperidone decreased the strength and frequency of abnormal information flow at high gamma and high frequencies while limiting mPFC → dHPC delta signals. Haloperidol's effects on phase coherence and signal directionality were comparable to those of the saline control group, except for mPFC → dHPC delta signals, which were prolonged in time. Modified from [13].

Both the PFC and HPC are densely innervated by axons from serotonin-producing neurons located in the dorsal and medial raphe nuclei, and they express both receptor types abundantly. In contrast, dopamine D2 receptors (D2Rs) are present at moderate levels in these regions, compared to the high densities found in other brain areas [32–36]. To gain further insight into the serotonergic component of atypical APDs, we investigated the efficacy of the 5-HT_{2A}R antagonist M100907 (1 mg/kg, i.p.) and the 5-HT_{1A}R agonist 8-OH-DPAT (1 mg/kg, i.p.) in reversing PCP-induced effects.

M100907 attenuated PCP-induced changes in both high- and middle-frequency bands (theta, alpha) in the mPFC, although delta and gamma bands remained

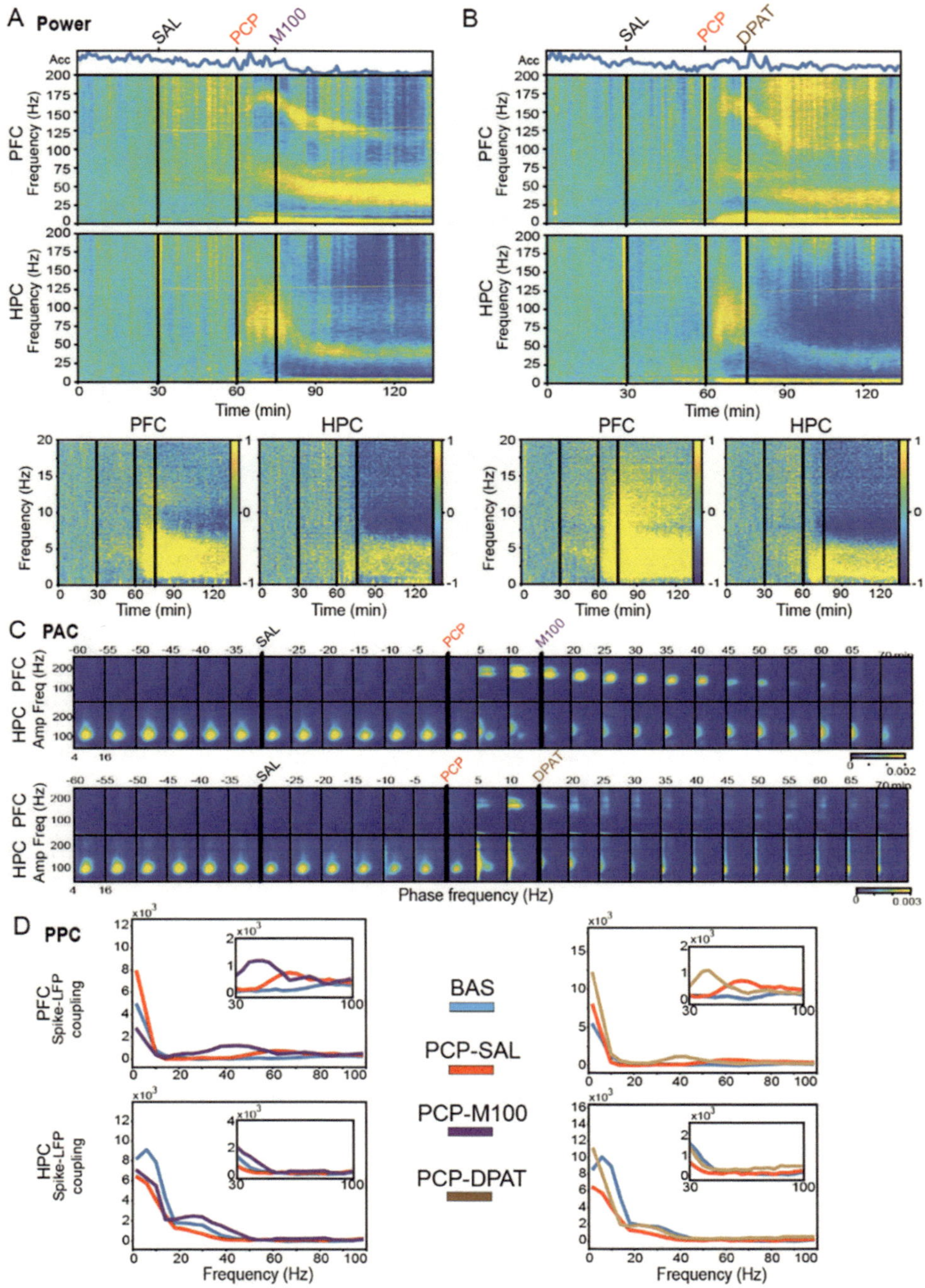

Figure 5.
Effects of the 5-HT$_{2A}$R antagonist M100907 and the 5-HT$_{1A}$R agonist 8-OH-DPAT on mPFC and dHPC neural activity during PCP-induced psychosis. (A) M100907 markedly reduced the power of aberrant theta, alpha, and high-frequency bands in the mPFC but was unable to diminish delta and gamma bands or restore hippocampal inhibition. Z-scores relative to baseline are shown. (B) 8-OH-DPAT showed limited efficacy compared to M100907 in attenuating PCP-induced effects. In fact, cortical high-frequency oscillations and hippocampal inhibition were exacerbated. (C) Both compounds effectively suppressed abnormal delta-high frequency coupling in the mPFC and preserved intra-hippocampal delta-gamma coupling, which was not observed with APDs. (D) Both M100907 and 8-OH-DPAT shifted cortical spike-LFP coupling toward slower gamma frequencies, consistent with changes seen in power bands. Modified from [13].

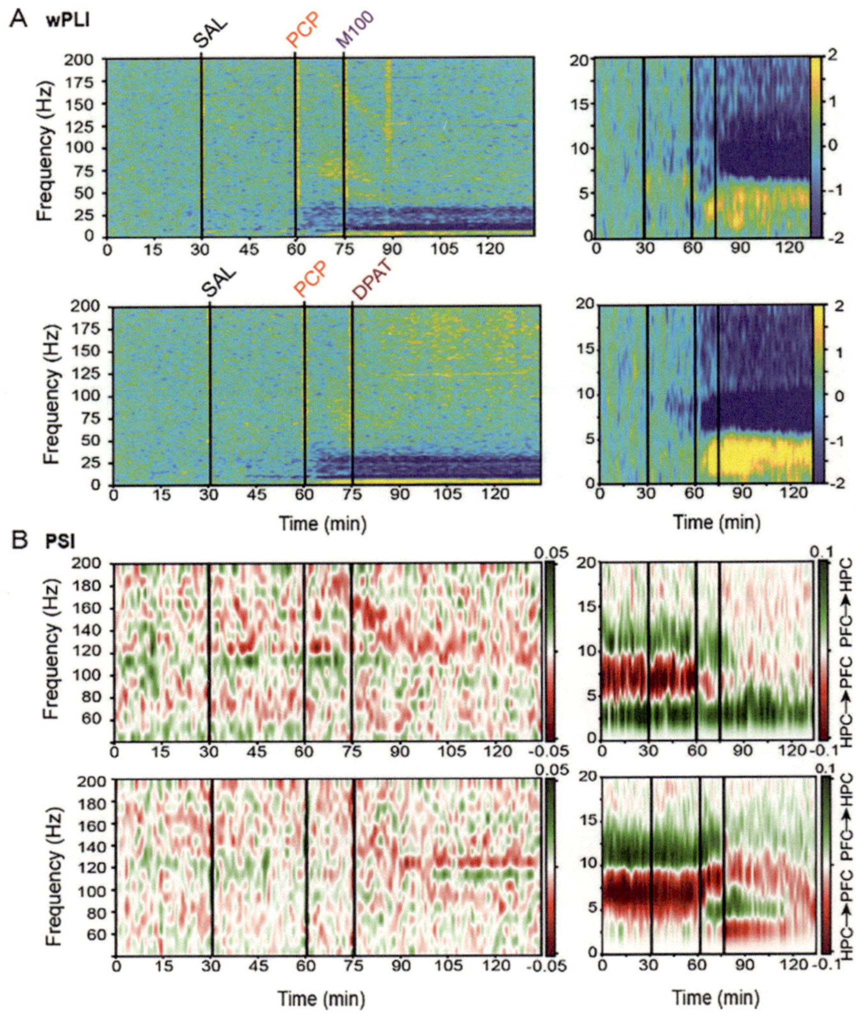

Figure 6.

Effects of M100907 and 8-OH-DPAT on mPFC-dHPC connectivity during PCP-induced psychosis. (A) Both compounds significantly reduced PCP-generated phase synchronization at gamma and high frequencies, with partial restoration of theta, alpha, and beta suppression. M100907 also attenuated aberrant delta coherence. Z-scores are shown relative to baseline. (B) Both compounds effectively reduced aberrant dHPC → mPFC gamma and high-frequency signals but failed to restore intrinsic theta connectivity. Modified from [13].

augmented. As with the APDs, the power of most oscillatory bands remained low in the dHPC. 8-OH-DPAT was less effective than M100907 in mitigating PCP-induced effects. In fact, cortical high-frequency oscillations and hippocampal inhibition were exacerbated compared to PCP alone. Both drugs, however, were highly effective in suppressing abnormal delta-high frequency coupling in the mPFC. In addition, while they did not fully restore intrinsic hippocampal theta-gamma coupling, some delta-gamma coupling remained. This suggests that the serotonin agents partially mitigated PCP-induced alterations in hippocampal neural network activity, a phenomenon not observed with APDs. In addition, both drugs also reduced the neuronal firing rates in both brain structures, and cortical spike-LFP coupling shifted to slower frequencies, closely following changes in oscillatory power (**Figure 5**).

At the circuit level, both M100907 and 8-OH-DPAT demonstrated superior efficacy compared to risperidone. They significantly reduced excessive phase synchronization and information flow at gamma and high frequencies, while partially restoring coherence in the theta, alpha, and beta bands. M100907 also attenuated aberrant mPFC → dHPC delta signals. However, neither compound succeeded in restoring the intrinsic dHPC → mPFC theta coordination (**Figure 6**).

Overall, the serotonergic compounds effectively normalized several power bands and phase-amplitude coupling in the mPFC, while partially restoring circuit connectivity. These findings suggest that 5-HT_{2A}R antagonism and 5-HT_{1A}R agonism play a role in modulating prefrontal-hippocampal pathways during psychotic-like states. Furthermore, they highlight the potential contribution of these mechanisms to the antipsychotic effects of atypical APDs such as risperidone and clozapine.

3. Neural substrates of cognitive impairment in a mouse model of schizophrenia

3.1 The phencyclidine model of cognitive impairment in schizophrenia

Chronic and subchronic administration of PCP to rodents induces prolonged cognitive impairments, lasting several weeks, and serves as a well-established model for studying the cognitive symptoms of schizophrenia [19, 20, 37]. In our studies, we utilized a subchronic PCP (sPCP) administration protocol involving two consecutive weeks of daily injections (Monday to Friday; 10 injections at 10 mg/kg, s.c.) to induce cognitive deficits persisting for at least 8 weeks. This duration was deemed reasonable to maintain high-quality electrophysiological signals for subsequent analyses. To validate our protocol, we evaluated memory performance in mice weekly over a 10-week period, excluding the initial recovery week following electrode implantation surgery. Signal quality was verified through analyses of oscillatory power and action potentials, ensuring high signal-to-noise ratios. With the model validated under our conditions, we examined the neural correlates of sPCP-induced deficits in recognition memory and auditory processing, as well as their potential reversal by risperidone (0.5 mg/kg, i.p, administered daily for 2 weeks). Across baseline (weeks 1 and 2), post-sPCP (weeks 5 and 6), and post-risperidone (weeks 9 and 10) phases, we combined behavioral assays with electrophysiological recordings conducted during the open field test, novel object recognition test (NOR), and two auditory tests—auditory evoked potentials (AEPs) and mismatch negativity (MMN) (**Figure 7**).

Short- and long-term recognition memories (STM and LTM, respectively) were evaluated using the NOR test, which leverages mice's innate preference for exploring novel over familiar objects in the environment. This behavior is strongly dependent on the HPC and recent studies, including our own, indeed suggest the involvement of hippocampal-prefrontal circuits [12, 38]. For these studies, we designed two custom T-mazes optimized for electrophysiological recordings. The mazes were constructed from aluminum, featuring wider and taller arms compared to standard designs, were grounded, and mounted on aluminum platforms to minimize noise interference [12, 14, 15]. Recognition memory performance was assessed under three experimental conditions: baseline (treatment-free), following sPCP administration, and after risperidone treatment. Consistent with prior research, mice displayed positive discrimination indices (DIs) for novel versus familiar objects during baseline testing in both the 3-minute (STM) and 24-hour (LTM) intervals, indicating intact recognition

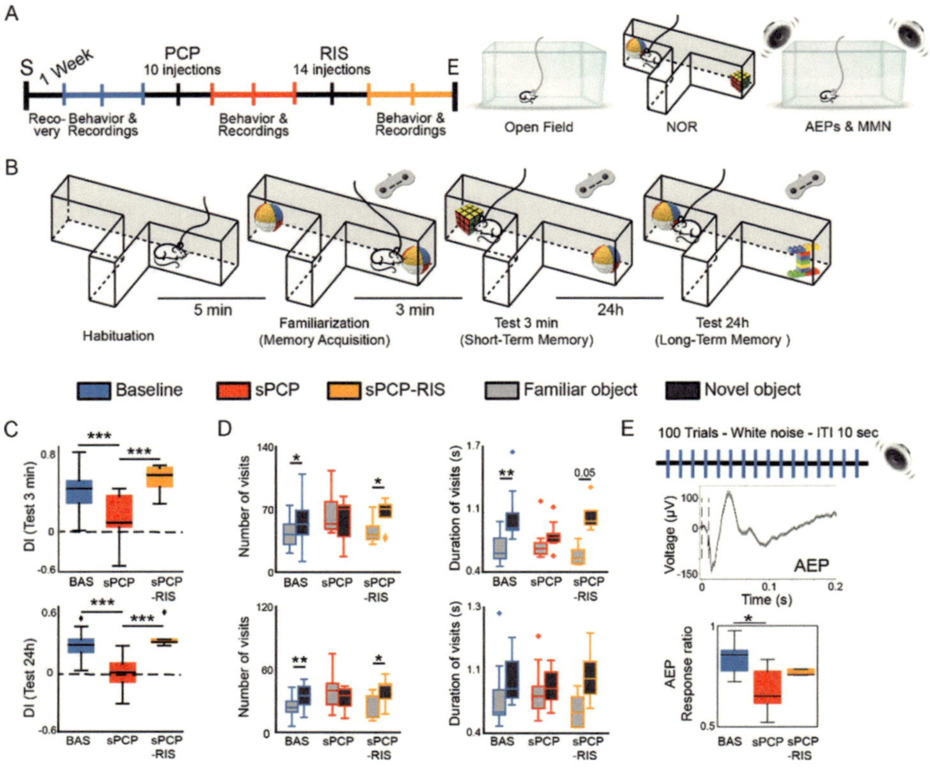

Figure 7.
sPCP-induced memory and auditory deficits reversed by risperidone. (A) Schematic of the experimental timeline and behavioral tests. S indicates surgery, and E indicates euthanasia. (B) The NOR task involved a habituation phase (exploration of the maze without objects), a familiarization phase (two identical objects placed in the maze), and short-term memory (STM) and long-term memory (LTM) tests with a familiar and a novel object. Each phase lasted 10 minutes, with STM and LTM tests conducted 3 minutes and 24 hours post-familiarization, respectively. (C) Discrimination indices (DIs) (calculated as [time visiting the novel object – time visiting the familiar object]/total exploration time) revealed significant memory impairments induced by sPCP that were rescued by risperidone. (D) In both STM and LTM tests, untreated animals showed a clear preference for the novel object, with increased exploration frequency and duration. This preference was lost in sPCP-treated mice but restored following risperidone treatment. (E) Auditory evoked potentials (AEPs) were assessed by measuring the ratio of responses in the mPFC to auditory stimuli. sPCP-treated mice exhibited reduced AEP ratios, which were partially restored by risperidone. Adapted from [14].

memory at the start of the experiments. However, sPCP treatment disrupted this behavior, as mice explored novel and familiar objects equally, reflecting impaired recognition memory. Notably, this deficit was reversed by risperidone treatment but not by saline (**Figure** 7 and **Table 3**).

Auditory processing and auditory attention were evaluated through auditory evoked potentials (AEPs) and mismatch negativity (MMN), respectively, under baseline, sPCP, and risperidone conditions. Both AEPs and MMN are highly translational biomarkers that have been extensively studied in patients and rodent models of schizophrenia, making them valuable tools in clinical and preclinical research [39–43]. To examine alterations in AEPs, mice were exposed to 100 auditory stimuli consisting of 15-millisecond white noise clicks. Within the same recording session, MMN was assessed using a passive oddball paradigm. MMN, a component of event-related potentials, reflects pre-attentive auditory sensory memory and is evoked by deviant auditory stimuli. This phenomenon has been well characterized in patients with schizophrenia.

		sPCP	Risperidone
Quiet alertness	mPFC	Increased high gamma power	Fully rescued
	dHPC	Decreased high gamma power and theta-gamma coupling	Coupling partially rescued
Memory acquisition	BEHAV	—	—
	mPFC	Increased theta power	Not rescued
	dHPC	Decreased high gamma power and theta-gamma coupling	Coupling partially rescued
	PSI	Disrupted mPFC → dHPC high gamma signals during familiar visits	Not rescued
Short-term memory	BEHAV	Decreased discrimination index	Fully rescued
	mPFC	Increased theta power	Not rescued
	dHPC	Decreased high gamma power and theta-gamma coupling	Partially rescued
	PSI	Disrupted mPFC → dHPC high gamma signals during familiar visits	Not rescued
Long-term memory	BEHAV.	Decreased discrimination index	Fully rescued
	mPFC	—	—
	dHPC	Decreased high gamma power and theta-gamma coupling	Partially rescued
	PSI	Disrupted dHPC → mPFC theta signals during familiar visits	Not rescued
Auditory processing	BEHAV.	Decreased response ratio	Partially rescued
	mPFC-P2	Decreased spiking activity	Partially rescued
	mPFC-P3	Decreased amplitude and spiking activity	Partially rescued
	MMN	MMN not present	Not rescued

Table 3.
Summary of main behavioral and neurophysiological results during baseline, sPCP and chronic risperidone conditions.

In our study, mice were presented with 1000 tones differing in frequency (6 kHz or 8 kHz), arranged in blocks with 25% target and 75% standard stimuli. After 500 trials, the standard and target frequencies were switched [44]. Neural activities were recorded in both the mPFC and the dHPC. However, hippocampal responses were inconsistent and highly variable across animals, leading us to focus on mPFC data. During baseline, cortical AEPs were detected in 82.3% of trials (response ratio: AEPs/total trials). Following sPCP administration, the response ratio decreased significantly to 64.7%, but partial recovery was observed with risperidone, increasing the response ratio to 71.8% (**Figure** 7 and **Table 3**). At baseline, MMN was observed during the 6–8 kHz target-standard tone combination, as indicated by a significant voltage difference between target and standard evoked potentials. However, MMN was not detected with the 8–6 kHz combination. After sPCP treatment, MMN was completely abolished and did not reappear following risperidone administration (see [14]).

Overall, while risperidone rescued sPCP-induced behavioral and neurophysiological disruptions in AEPs, it failed to restore MMN responses. These findings may indicate differential impact of risperidone on auditory processing versus auditory attention deficits.

3.2 Natural synchronization of prefrontal-hippocampal circuits during quiet alertness and recognition memory

The PFC and HPC exhibit strong synchronized activity during active cognitive engagement. This natural synchronization is particularly prominent in the theta frequency range (4–12 Hz), which facilitates communication between these regions and supports memory encoding and retrieval. We collected an extensive dataset of local and circuit-level neural signals from over 20 mice during periods of quiet alertness and throughout the three phases of the NOR test. To minimize confounding effects of hyperlocomotion induced by sPCP treatment [19, 45], our initial analyses focused on neural activity during resting states. These were defined as brief, 3-second episodes of minimal behavioral activity observed while the untreated mice explored an open field. As expected, during resting states, mice exhibited pronounced circuit synchronization at theta frequencies (4–12 Hz). Theta oscillations were prominent in the mPFC and were accompanied by robust theta oscillations, theta-gamma coupling, and spike-theta coupling in the dHPC. Interestingly, despite the observed local theta synchronization during these brief quiet periods, the phase coherence and directionality of signals within the mPFC-dHPC circuit appeared to be notably weak.

To account for the sensitivity of certain mathematical tools to time window selection, we concatenated consecutive visits during the NOR task until the accumulated duration reached 5 seconds. This approach allowed for direct comparisons of neural activity across different behaviors, such as visits to familiar and novel objects. However, spike-LFP coupling could not be reliably estimated due to an insufficient number of action potentials for accurate calculations (for details, see [14]). Memory acquisition was analyzed by comparing neural signals recorded during the first and last visits to the two identical objects in the familiarization phase (the first 5 seconds versus the last 5 seconds of visits to either object). Results indicated that memory acquisition was associated with increased theta power in the mPFC, decreased theta and gamma power in the dHPC, and enhanced high-gamma signals propagating from the mPFC to the dHPC (mPFC → dHPC). That is, these effects were more pronounced during late visits compared to early visits.

Short-term and long-term memory retrieval were assessed by comparing neurophysiological signals recorded during the first 5 seconds of visits to novel objects versus the first 5 seconds of visits to familiar objects in the 3-minute (STM) and 24-hour (LTM) tests. Notably, no differences in power or theta-gamma coupling were observed between visits to novel and familiar objects in either region during either test. However, directional high-gamma signals from the mPFC to the dHPC were detected during visits to familiar objects in the STM test, similar to the patterns observed during memory acquisition. In contrast, theta signals propagating from the dHPC to the mPFC emerged during visits to familiar objects in the LTM test. These directional signal patterns appeared to be relevant for memory processing, as they exhibited strong correlations with memory performance (Pearson's $R = 0.7$, DI with high-gamma PSI for STM; $R = -0.72$, DI with theta PSI for LTM). This underscores the importance of specific oscillatory dynamics and inter-regional communication in supporting different phases of recognition memory.

Together, these findings highlight the contribution of theta and gamma connectivity signals within mPFC-dHPC circuits to normal memory acquisition, as well as short-term and long-term memory processes, in the context of object recognition. The observed flow of information between these regions likely plays a critical role in supporting these cognitive functions.

3.3 Prefrontal-hippocampal circuits during sPCP-induced cognitive impairments and partial rescue by risperidone

sPCP administration increased theta power in prefrontal microcircuits and disrupted high gamma rhythms and theta-gamma coupling in the dHPC across various brain states and memory tasks. These neurophysiological alterations were consistently observed across different experimental days. Notably, the chronic administration of risperidone partially alleviated some of these disruptions, hippocampal gamma oscillations and theta-gamma coupling in a more consistent manner, suggesting a preferential effect on the dHPC. In contrast, risperidone had minimal influence on the circuit's connectivity (PSI). These findings suggest that the chronic administration of risperidone may improve cognitive functions through its effects on hippocampal microcircuits in schizophrenia patients. A detailed summary of the study's results is presented in **Table 3**.

4. Conclusions

- PCP-induced psychosis enhanced prefrontal synchronization, disrupted hippocampal synchrony, and impaired circuit connectivity. A pathological delta synchronization emerged locally and across the circuit.

- During PCP-induced psychosis, risperidone alleviated cortical disturbances with minimal impact on the dHPC, whereas haloperidol exacerbated circuit disruptions, revealing distinct effects of atypical and classical APDs on prefrontal-hippocampal dynamics.

- 5-HT_{2A}R antagonism and 5-HT_{1A}R agonism outperformed risperidone in restoring prefrontal-hippocampal dynamics, highlighting the serotonin system as a target for alleviating psychosis-related pathophysiological alterations.

- Subchronic PCP administration increased theta power in prefrontal microcircuits and disrupted theta-gamma synchronization in the dHPC across diverse brain states and memory tasks.

- Chronic risperidone treatment influenced hippocampal microcircuits, providing a neural framework for its cognitive benefits in schizophrenia.

Acknowledgements

We thank Drs. Maria Alemany-González and Cristina Delgado-Sallent, as well as Mr. Pau Nebot, for their invaluable contribution to this work. This work was funded by grants PID2019-104683RB-I00 and PID2022-139089OB-I00 funded by MCIN/AEI/10.13039/501100011033/ and by FEDER A way of making Europe.

Conflict of interest

The authors declare no conflict of interest.

Author details

Maria Victoria Puig*, Thomas Gener, Cristina López-Cabezón and Sara Hidalgo-Nieves
Institute of Biomedical Research of Barcelona, CSIC, Barcelona, Spain

*Address all correspondence to: victoria.puig@iibb.csic.es

References

[1] Gonzalez-Burgos G, Cho RY, Lewis DA. Alterations in cortical network oscillations and parvalbumin neurons in schizophrenia. Biological Psychiatry. 2015;**77**:1031-1040. DOI: 10.1016/j.biopsych.2015.03.010

[2] Goldman AL, Pezawas L, Doz P, Mattay VS, Fischl B, Verchinski BA, et al. Widespread reductions of cortical thickness in schizophrenia and spectrum disorders and evidence of heritability. Archives of General Psychiatry. 2009;**66**:467. DOI: 10.1001/archgenpsychiatry.2009.24

[3] Miller EK, Cohen JD. An integrative theory of prefrontal cortex function. Annual Review of Neuroscience. 2001;**24**:167-202. DOI: 10.1146/annurev.neuro.24.1.167

[4] Uhlhaas PJ, Singer W. Abnormal neural oscillations and synchrony in schizophrenia. Nature Reviews. Neuroscience. 2010;**11**:100-113. DOI: 10.1038/nrn2774

[5] Behrendt RP, Young C. Hallucinations in schizophrenia, sensory impairment, and brain disease: A unifying model. The Behavioral and Brain Sciences. 2004;**27**:771-787. DOI: 10.1017/s0140525x04000184

[6] Spencer KM, Nestor PG, Niznikiewicz MA, Salisbury DF, Shenton ME, McCarley RW. Abnormal neural synchrony in schizophrenia. The Journal of Neuroscience. 2003;**23**:7407-7411. DOI: 10.1523/JNEUROSCI.23-19-07407.2003

[7] Sun L, Castellanos N, Grützner C, Koethe D, Rivolta D, Wibral M, et al. Evidence for dysregulated high-frequency oscillations during sensory processing in medication-naïve, first episode schizophrenia. Schizophrenia Research. 2013;**150**:519-525. DOI: 10.1016/j.schres.2013.08.023

[8] Grützner C, Wibral M, Sun L, Rivolta D, Singer W, Maurer K, et al. Deficits in high- (>60 Hz) gamma-band oscillations during visual processing in schizophrenia. Frontiers in Human Neuroscience. 2013;**7**:88. DOI: 10.3389/fnhum.2013.00088

[9] Sigurdsson T, Stark KL, Karayiorgou M, Gogos JA, Gordon JA. Impaired hippocampal–prefrontal synchrony in a genetic mouse model of schizophrenia. Nature. 2010;**464**:763-767. DOI: 10.1038/nature08855

[10] Sigurdsson T, Duvarci S. Hippocampal-prefrontal interactions in cognition, behavior and psychiatric disease. Frontiers in Systems Neuroscience. 2016;**9**:190. DOI: 10.3389/fnsys.2015.00190

[11] Gener T, Tauste Campo A, Alemany-González M, Nebot P, Delgado-Sallent C, Chanovas J, et al. Serotonin 5-HT1A, 5-HT2A and dopamine D2 receptors strongly influence prefronto-hippocampal neural networks in alert mice: Contribution to the actions of risperidone. Neuropharmacology. 2019;**158**:107743. DOI: 10.1016/j.neuropharm.2019.107743

[12] Alemany-González M, Gener T, Nebot P, Vilademunt M, Dierssen M, Puig MV. Prefrontal-hippocampal functional connectivity encodes recognition memory and is impaired in intellectual disability. Proceedings of the National Academy of Sciences of the United States of America. 2020;**117**:11788-11798. DOI: 10.1073/pnas.1921314117

[13] Delgado-Sallent C, Nebot P, Gener T, Fath AB, Timplalexi M, Puig MV. Atypical, but not typical, antipsychotic drugs reduce hypersynchronized prefrontal-hippocampal circuits during psychosis-like states in mice: Contribution of 5-HT2A and 5-HT1A receptors. Cerebral Cortex. 2022;**32**:3472-3487. DOI: 10.1093/cercor/bhab427

[14] Delgado-Sallent C, Gener T, Nebot P, López-Cabezón C, Puig MV. Neural substrates of cognitive impairment in a NMDAR hypofunction mouse model of schizophrenia and partial rescue by risperidone. Frontiers in Cellular Neuroscience. 2023;**17**:1152248. DOI: 10.3389/fncel.2023.1152248

[15] Alemany-González M, Vilademunt M, Gener T, Puig MV. Postnatal environmental enrichment enhances memory through distinct neural mechanisms in healthy and trisomic female mice. Neurobiology of Disease. 2022;**173**:105841. DOI: 10.1016/j.nbd.2022.105841

[16] Krystal JH, Karper LP, Seibyl JP, Freeman GK, Delaney R, Bremner JD, et al. Subanesthetic effects of the noncompetitive NMDA antagonist, ketamine, in humans. Psychotomimetic, perceptual, cognitive, and neuroendocrine responses. Archives of General Psychiatry. 1994;**51**:199-214. DOI: 10.1001/archpsyc.1994.03950030035004

[17] Lahti AC, Koffel B, LaPorte D, Tamminga CA. Subanesthetic doses of ketamine stimulate psychosis in schizophrenia. Neuropsychopharmacology. 1995;**13**:9-19. DOI: 10.1016/0893-133X(94)00131-I

[18] Sturgeon RD, Fessler RG, Meltzer HY. Behavioral rating scales for assessing phencyclidine-induced locomotor activity, stereotyped behavior and ataxia in rats. European Journal of Pharmacology. 1979;**16**(59):169-179. DOI: 10.1016/0014-2999(79)90279-6

[19] Castañé A, Santana N, Artigas F. PCP-based mice models of schizophrenia: Differential behavioral, neurochemical and cellular effects of acute and subchronic treatments. Psychopharmacology. 2015;**232**:4085-4097. DOI: 10.1007/s00213-015-3946-6

[20] Meltzer HY, Rajagopal L, Huang M, Oyamada Y, Kwon S, Horiguchi M. Translating the N-methyl-d-aspartate receptor antagonist model of schizophrenia to treatments for cognitive impairment in schizophrenia. International Journal of Neuropsychopharmacology. 2013;**16**:2181-2194. DOI: 10.1017/S1461145713000928

[21] He BJ. Scale-free brain activity: Past, present, and future. Trends in Cognitive Sciences. 2014;**18**:480-487. DOI: 10.1016/j.tics.2014.04.003

[22] Scheffer-Teixeira R, Tort ABL. Unveiling fast field oscillations through comodulation. eNeuro. 2017;**4**:ENEURO.0079-17.2017. DOI: 10.1523/ENEURO.0079-17.2017

[23] Vinck M, Battaglia FP, Womelsdorf T, Pennartz C. Improved measures of phase-coupling between spikes and the local field potential. Journal of Computational Neuroscience. 2012;**33**:53-75. DOI: 10.1007/s10827-011-0374-4

[24] Vinck M, Oostenveld R, van Wingerden M, Battaglia F, Pennartz CMA. An improved index of phase-synchronization for electrophysiological data in the presence of volume-conduction, noise and sample-size bias. NeuroImage.

2011;**55**:1548-1565. DOI: 10.1016/j.neuroimage.2011.01.055

[25] Nolte G, Ziehe A, Nikulin VV, Schlögl A, Krämer N, Brismar T, et al. Robustly estimating the flow direction of information in complex physical systems. Physical Review Letters. 2008;**100**:234101. DOI: 10.1103/PhysRevLett.100.234101

[26] Buzsáki G. Theta oscillations in the hippocampus. Neuron. 2002;**33**(3):325-340. DOI: 10.1016/s0896-6273(02)00586-x

[27] Borderie A, Caclin A, Lachaux JP, Perrone-Bertollotti M, Hoyer RS, Kahane P, et al. Cross-frequency coupling in cortico-hippocampal networks supports the maintenance of sequential auditory information in short-term memory. PLoS Biology. 2024;**22**:e3002512. DOI: 10.1371/journal.pbio.3002512

[28] Amour S, di Chanaz L, Pérez-Bellido A, Wu X, Lozano-Soldevilla D, Pacheco-Estefan D, et al. Gamma amplitude is coupled to opposed hippocampal theta-phase states during the encoding and retrieval of episodic memories in humans. Current Biology. 2023;**33**:1836-1843.e6. DOI: 10.1016/j.cub.2023.03.073

[29] Vivekananda U, Bush D, Bisby JA, Baxendale S, Rodionov R, Diehl B, et al. Theta power and theta-gamma coupling support long-term spatial memory retrieval. Hippocampus. 2021;**31**:213-220. DOI: 10.1002/hipo.23284

[30] Colgin LL. Theta-gamma coupling in the entorhinal-hippocampal system. Current Opinion in Neurobiology. 2015;**31**:45-50. DOI: 10.1016/j.conb.2014.08.001

[31] Meltzer H, Massey B. The role of serotonin receptors in the action of atypical antipsychotic drugs. Current Opinion in Pharmacology. 2011;**11**:59-67. DOI: 2014-11-20 14:20:38

[32] Celada P, Puig MV, Artigas F. Serotonin modulation of cortical neurons and networks. Frontiers in Integrative Neuroscience. 2013;7:25. DOI: 10.3389/fnint.2013.00025

[33] Puig MV, Gulledge AT. Serotonin and prefrontal cortex function: Neurons, networks, and circuits. Molecular Neurobiology. 2011;**44**:449-464. DOI: 10.1007/s12035-011-8214-0

[34] Berumen LC, Rodríguez A, Miledi R, García-Alcocer G. Serotonin receptors in hippocampus. The Scientific World Journal. 2012;**2012**:823493 DOI: 10.1100/2012/823493

[35] Puig MV, Gener T. Serotonin modulation of prefronto-hippocampal rhythms in health and disease. ACS Chemical Neuroscience. 2015;**6**:1017-1025. DOI: 10.1021/cn500350e

[36] Santana N, Mengod G, Artigas F. Quantitative analysis of the expression of dopamine D1 and D2 receptors in pyramidal and GABAergic neurons of the rat prefrontal cortex. Cerebral Cortex. 2009;**19**:849-860. DOI: 10.1093/cercor/bhn134

[37] Meltzer HY, Horiguchi M, Massey BW. The role of serotonin in the NMDA receptor antagonist models of psychosis and cognitive impairment. Psychopharmacology. 2011;**213**:289-305. DOI: 10.1007/s00213-010-2137-8

[38] Warburton EC, Brown MW. Neural circuitry for rat recognition memory. Behavioural Brain Research. 2015;**285**:131-139. DOI: 10.1016/j.bbr.2014.09.050

[39] Amann LC, Gandal MJ, Halene TB, Ehrlichman RS, White SL, McCarren HS,

et al. Mouse behavioral endophenotypes for schizophrenia. Brain Research Bulletin. 2010;**83**:147-161. DOI: 10.1016/j.brainresbull.2010.04.008

[40] Nagai T, Tada M, Kirihara K, Araki T, Jinde S, Kasai K. Mismatch negativity as a "translatable" brain marker toward early intervention for psychosis: A review. Frontiers in Psychiatry. 2013;**4**:115. DOI: 10.3389/fpsyt.2013.00115

[41] Javitt DC, Sweet RA. Auditory dysfunction in schizophrenia: Integrating clinical and basic features. Nature Reviews. Neuroscience. 2015;**16**:535-550. DOI: 10.1038/nrn4002

[42] Modi ME, Sahin M. Translational use of event-related potentials to assess circuit integrity in ASD. Nature Reviews. Neurology. 2017;**13**:160-170. DOI: 10.1038/nrneurol.2017.15

[43] Viana D, Walston ST, Masvidal-Codina E, Illa X, Rodríguez-Meana B, Del Valle J, et al. Nanoporous graphene-based thin-film microelectrodes for in vivo high-resolution neural recording and stimulation. Nature Nanotechnology. 2024;**19**:514-523. DOI: 10.1038/s41565-023-01570-5

[44] Hamilton HK, Perez VB, Ford JM, Roach BJ, Jaeger J, Mathalon DH. Mismatch negativity but not P300 is associated with functional disability in schizophrenia. Schizophrenia Bulletin. 2018;**44**:492-504. DOI: 10.1093/schbul/sbx104

[45] Mouri A, Koseki T, Narusawa S, Niwa M, Mamiya T, Kano SI, et al. Mouse strain differences in phencyclidine-induced behavioural changes. The International Journal of Neuropsychopharmacology. 2012;**15**:767-779. DOI: 10.1017/S146114571100085X

Chapter 4

Perspective Chapter: The Neuropsychological Dimension of Psychosis – Implications for Assessment and Treatment

Sotiria Moza and Savvina Chrysostomou

Abstract

Psychotic Spectrum Disorders (PSDs) affect approximately 1 in 300 people worldwide and encompass a range of positive symptoms, such as hallucinations, delusions, and disorganized thinking, as well as negative symptoms, including alogia, avolition, and diminished emotional expression. In addition, people with PSDs frequently present impairments in cognitive domains, such as executive function, memory, attention, and social cognition, which lead to difficulties in independent living, employment, and interpersonal relationships. This chapter explores the neuropsychological dimension of psychosis and provides a thorough summary of the cognitive deficits linked to PSDs. The neurobiological underpinnings of these impairments are discussed, examining PSD differentiations in brain structure and function. Instruments used for neuropsychological evaluation in PSDs are presented, supporting the crucial role formal evaluation plays in diagnosis and treatment. Modern therapeutic modalities, such as cognitive remediation therapies, pharmaceutical interventions, and technologies like neurostimulation and digital therapeutics, are discussed. The chapter closes by discussing implications for future study and clinical application, highlighting the necessity of integrated, culturally relevant, and ethical approaches for cognitive rehabilitation and symptom management. Through this work, the authors aim to support a better understanding of psychosis and promote more efficient, comprehensive care for people with PSDs.

Keywords: psychosis, PSD, neuropsychology, assessment, cognitive remediation, neuropsychological rehabilitation, treatment outcomes, ADLs, activities of daily living

1. Introduction

Schizophrenia and other psychotic disorders impact a large percentage of the world's population. One of the most common psychotic diseases, schizophrenia, affects about 24 million people globally, or roughly 1 in 300 people and 1 in 222 adults [1]. Other psychotic diseases vary in prevalence. For instance, the median lifetime prevalence for probable psychosis was 17.24 per 1000 people, 8.8 per 1000 for schizophrenia and related disorders, 8.18 per 1000 for non-affective psychosis, and 6.35 per 1000 for schizophrenia alone, according to a systematic study performed in 2018 [2].

A framework for understanding and diagnosing psychotic disorders is provided by the DSM-5 [3, 4]. According to the criteria, psychosis has five dimensions, namely, (a) delusions, which include persistent, unprovable erroneous beliefs that are impervious to proof, such as grandiose (belief in extraordinary talents) or persecutory (belief of being targeted), (b) hallucinations, which are perception-like experiences that are caused by abnormalities in sensory processing and are typically auditory in nature, (c) disorganized thinking, which manifests as speech irregularities such as loose associations or incoherence, (d) motor disruptions, highlighted by grossly disordered or aberrant motor behavior, such as catatonia, and spanning from unpredictable agitation to unresponsiveness, and (e) deficiencies in reward processing and emotional dysregulation which lead to a reduction or loss of typical functioning, such as motivation (avolition) or impaired emotional expressiveness (affective flattening). These symptoms, often experienced by individuals with Psychotic Spectrum Disorders (PSDs), are broadly categorized as positive and negative. Delusions, hallucinations, and disorganized thought patterns are examples of positive symptoms, so-called because they add to the person's reality and experience. Conversely, negative signs, such as social disengagement, avolition (lack of motivation), and alogia (limited speech), indicate a decrease or loss in normal functioning. Finally, the degree of psychosis, the number of symptoms, and the duration of psychosis remain in use as diagnostic elements distinguishing PSDs from each other [3, 4].

Numerous studies have consistently found that people with PSDs experience certain cognitive deficits that have a major influence on their day-to-day lives. These deficits most commonly affect working memory, executive functioning, attention, language, emotional regulation, and social cognition, and are closely linked to brain function [5, 6]. For example, delusions and hallucinations are often associated with impairments in reasoning and memory, particularly in attributing causality or processing reality-based evidence [5]. Likewise, these symptoms may be associated with disruptions in sensory processing and integration, as well as heightened activity in regions such as the auditory cortex [6]. In addition, disorganized thinking, such as speech derailment, may indicate impairments in executive function, working memory, and language processing, as well as abnormal activity in the prefrontal cortex and anterior cingulate cortex [5]. Moreover, negative symptoms such as avolition, anhedonia, and emotional flatness are often tied to deficits in reward processing, motivation, and emotional regulation, indicating dysfunction in brain areas such as the ventral striatum and prefrontal cortex. Finally, abnormal motor behavior, such as agitation and catatonia, may be associated with deficits in motor planning, control, and integration, potentially linked to frontal lobe dysfunction [7].

These cognitive deficits and their structural and functional brain correlates are not only of scientific interest but also have significant implications for the everyday life capabilities of people with PSDs, including employment, relationships, and education, thereby making them crucial for designing psychosocial interventions. According to recent studies, an array of psychosocial and behavioral approaches, such as cognitive behavioral therapy, skills retraining, and neurostimulation therapies, hold promise for treating these symptoms. Among these, neuropsychological remediation therapy receives particular attention since it focuses on the basis of cognitive function, addressing skills that are most frequently impacted, including working memory, executive control, planning, attention, language, emotional regulation, and social cognition [8, 9]. This chapter aims to explore the neuropsychological dimension of psychosis, addressing the cognitive deficits associated with various psychosis profiles, their neurobiological underpinnings, and the tools used for assessment. Additionally, it examines the implications of these deficits for everyday functionality and discusses modern treatment approaches and emerging trends, as well as limitations in addressing these challenges in modern settings.

2. Psychosis from neuropsychological point of view

2.1 Psychosis and its clinical manifestation

Psychosis is a clinical syndrome characterized by a disruption in thought processes, perceptions, emotions, and overall behavior [10, 11]. These changes result in detachment from reality, rendering people unable to understand and respond to environmental stimuli [12, 13]. The presence of hallucinations, delusions, and disorganized thinking are required as clinical criteria to diagnose psychosis [14]. For more information, please see **Figure 1**.

Psychotic disorders are categorized based on their duration, severity, and functional impairments. In the Diagnostic and Statistical Manual of Mental Disorders, Fifth Edition (DSM-5) it is stated that psychotic symptoms can either arise in the form of psychiatric conditions such as schizophrenia or from other neurological and medical conditions or they can be substance-induced [15–17]. Moreover, the disorders in the psychotic spectrum have common symptoms as well as differences, especially in symptom expression and severity. Similarly, the International Classification of Diseases (ICD-11) describes psychosis as a syndrome with varying etiologies, emphasizing the need for comprehensive assessments that consider biological, psychological, and social factors [18].

Psychosis is a mental condition marked by a significant loss of contact with reality, typically impacting five key domains categorized in positive and negative symptoms as well as, daily functioning and overall quality of life.

Positive Symptoms (Distortion of normal function)

- Hallucinations (sensory perceptions without external stimuli present)
- Delusions (false beliefs including paranoia)
- Disorganized thinking (incoherent and fragmented speech and thoughts)
- Abnormal motor behavior (agitation, catatonia, purposeless movements)

Negative Symptoms (Reduction/loss of normal function)

- Affective flattening (Reduced emotional expression, characterized by a lack of variation in tone of speech and minimal facial expressions)
- Alogia (reduced verbal communication)
- Anhedonia (reduced capacity of receiving pleasure)
- Avolition (lack of motivation and action initiation)
- Social withdrawal (lack of engagement and reduced social interactions)

Figure 1.
Psychosis definition and symptom overview.

2.2 Overview of neuropsychological deficits in psychosis

Several previous studies have indicated that psychosis is associated with neurobiological and neuropsychological impairments. Neuroimaging studies have indicated that certain areas of the brain, such as the prefrontal cortex, hippocampus, and amygdala, are altered in PSDs [11, 19, 20]. These areas play an important role in executive function, memory, and emotional regulation. As a result, impairments in attention, working memory, and decision-making are commonly noted among individuals with psychotic symptoms [11, 21, 22].

Deficits in working memory and attention are among the most common symptoms of psychosis. Impaired working memory makes it difficult to process, store temporarily, and mentally manipulate information, which can severely limit the ability to plan, reason, and solve problems, as well as to communicate and maintain interpersonal relationships. In addition, attention deficits are pronounced among people with PSDs. The ability to focus on important stimuli and block out distractions is particularly affected, which often leads to significant difficulties in thinking and performing everyday tasks [23, 24].

Moreover, executive function, which involves the ability to plan, organize, initiate, monitor, and even inhibit behavior and actions, is another cognitive domain which seems to be particularly sensitive in psychosis. Deficits in executive function are associated with poor social and occupational outcomes, as individuals struggle with tasks that require goal-directed behavior, problem-solving, and adaptive functioning [25, 26]. These deficits are often observed in conjunction with other cognitive impairments, such as difficulties in verbal fluency and reasoning [27]. Furthermore, impairments in executive function may be a key driver of negative symptoms in schizophrenia, such as apathy, lack of motivation, and social withdrawal [27–30].

Research indicates that neuropsychological differences in individuals with psychosis can vary across different age groups, including children, adolescents, young adults, and older adults depending on the age of onset of the psychosis.

Research has indicated that children with early-onset schizophrenia demonstrate lower performance in intelligence, memory, and perceptual motor skills tasks compared to groups with onset during adolescence and adulthood. Furthermore, adolescents showed greater difficulties in intelligence and memory than adults. These findings suggest that younger individuals with psychosis experience more pronounced cognitive impairments, potentially due to the disruption of critical developmental processes [31].

In Studies have shown that adolescents and young adults exhibit neuropsychological impairments, especially in verbal learning, sustained attention, and executive functioning, when compared to healthy individuals [31, 32]. Another longitudinal study showed that young adults with psychotic episodes had poorer mental health outcomes and functional difficulties as they transitioned into adulthood; a study supportive of the lifespan trajectory of psychosis. Specifically, they exhibited deficits in tasks requiring attention and processing speed, such as the Stroop Word-Color Test and the Purdue Pegboard, indicating early cognitive vulnerabilities that may persist into later life [33].

Moreover, older adults with psychotic experiences exhibit more pronounced cognitive impairments, particularly in measures of intelligence, working memory, and overall cognitive functioning compared to age-matched peers with no psychotic symptoms [34]. Finally, recent longitudinal studies have identified psychosis as a factor that differentiates dementia risk among older adults. This finding suggests that psychosis not only distinguishes individuals with PSDs from healthy controls but may also accelerate the cognitive decline associated with aging and dementia. Thus, current findings highlight the importance of psychosis as a critical clinical metric in assessing and managing cognitive health in older populations [35].

2.3 Neuropsychological profiles across psychotic disorders

Each psychotic disorder has unique neuropsychological patterns that reflect variations in their underlying neuropathology and disease course, even though some cognitive deficits are shared by all of them. In modern healthcare and clinical settings, it is essential to comprehend these profiles in order to customize interventions and develop treatment plans.

2.3.1 Schizophrenia spectrum disorders

The defining characteristic of Schizophrenia Spectrum Disorders (SCZ) is global cognitive impairments. Research has shown that people with SCZ usually score 1–2 standard deviations lower than healthy controls on the majority of neuropsychological tests [36] with memory, information processing speed, and executive functioning including inhibition, cognitive flexibility, and problem-solving being the main affected domains [36, 37]. People with schizophrenia frequently exhibit widespread difficulties in verbal and nonverbal memory, motor skills, attention, intellectual ability, spatial reasoning, executive functioning, and language abilities [38–40]. Finally, a neurodevelopmental trajectory is suggested by the evidence within the neuropsychological deficits in SCZ interpretation framework, with premorbid cognitive deficits appearing to worsen across the lifespan [41].

2.3.2 Bipolar disorder with psychotic symptoms

Although often less severe, neuropsychological deficits in bipolar disorder (BD) with psychotic characteristics are similar to those seen in SCZ. According to Mann-Wrobel and colleagues [42], deficits are particularly noticeable in executive functioning, memory, and processing speed. However, cognitive impairment in BD is very diverse, driven by the presence or absence of psychotic symptoms, history, and illness stage. More prominent deficits have been found among people with BD with psychotic features during the acute phases of the disorder which, however, seem to be reduced during remission from affective symptoms. Still, the methodological issues in this area of study, such as sample heterogeneity, limited sample numbers, and inadequate management of the impact of pharmaceutical treatment, affect the generalizability and consistency of the findings [42, 43].

2.3.3 Brief psychotic disorder

Brief Psychotic Disorder (BPD) is characterized by the presence of at least one positive psychotic symptom, such as non-bizarre delusions, hallucinations, disorganized speech, or markedly disorganized or catatonic behavior whose duration is less than a month with full recovery to the premorbid status. The diagnosis should not fit the criteria for schizophrenia, schizoaffective disorder, psychotic mood disorders, delusional disorder, acute psychotic disorder, schizophreniform disorder, or psychotic disorders caused by medical conditions or substance use [3].

Due to the relatively low prevalence of the disorder, there is limited research regarding the cognitive deficits associated with BPD. Studies on PSDs have reported deficits in executive functioning, memory, and attention as common in all disorders with psychotic characteristics [12]. Yet, the impairments associated with BPD are more likely to be resolved, by definition, upon the remittance of the disorder.

2.3.4 Substance-induced psychosis

Substance-induced psychosis (SIP) is also a relatively understudied disorder. Research shows that SIP-related cognitive deficits mimic the ones of core psychotic disorders. Executive functioning, memory, and attention are frequently impacted, mirroring deficiencies observed in core psychotic disorders while their magnitude is often comparable to schizophrenia. The diversity of these impairments is significantly influenced by substance-use parameters, including the type of substance, duration, and intensity of use, cessation patterns, and the extent of brain damage [44].

2.3.5 Comparative analysis of cognitive impairments

Although psychotic diseases share common cognitive deficits, especially regarding executive functioning, memory, and attention, the degree and persistence of these impairments differ widely between them. These variations highlight how crucial individualized evaluation and intervention techniques are in order to design effective treatment plans.

All results are summarized in **Table 1**.

3. Neurobiological underpinnings of psychosis

Research has shown that neuropsychological deficits in PSDs have a neurobiological foundation, with distinct structural and functional brain abnormalities consistently observed among individuals with psychosis.

3.1 Brain regions implicated in psychosis

Psychosis is closely associated with abnormalities in several critical brain regions, including the prefrontal cortex, hippocampus, thalamus, temporal lobes, and choroid plexus. Neuroimaging and neuropsychological studies consistently demonstrate structural and functional alterations in these areas, contributing to the cognitive and clinical symptoms characteristic of psychotic disorders.

Emerging research highlights the role of the choroid plexus, a structure responsible for producing cerebrospinal fluid (CSF), in psychosis. Enlarged choroid plexus volumes have been observed in individuals with psychotic disorders, correlating with reduced gray matter and poorer cognitive performance [45–47]. These findings suggest a potential neuro-immune mechanism underlying psychosis, linking structural changes in the choroid plexus to broader neurobiological disruptions. Furthermore, the thalamus, essential for cognitive processing, exhibits reduced volumes in psychotic disorders, with specific nuclei such as the pulvinar, closely associated with cognitive abilities [48–50]. These abnormalities are evident across populations, including both adults and youth with psychotic symptoms, emphasizing the thalamus's critical role in the neurodevelopmental trajectories. Moreover, the hippocampus, particularly

Psychotic disorder	Common cognitive impairments	Key findings	References
Schizophrenia Spectrum Disorders (SCZ)	Global cognitive impairments: memory, processing speed, executive functioning (inhibition, flexibility, problem-solving).	Premorbid cognitive deficits worsen over the lifespan. Widespread difficulties in verbal/nonverbal memory, motor skills, attention, spatial reasoning, and language abilities.	[36–41]
Bipolar Disorder with Psychotic Features (BD)	Executive functioning, memory, processing speed.	Deficits vary by illness stage and the presence of psychotic symptoms. More pronounced during acute phases, reduced in remission. Generalizability is affected by sample heterogeneity and pharmaceutical impacts.	[39, 43]
Brief Psychotic Disorder (BPD)	Executive functioning, memory, and attention (common to all psychotic disorders).	Impairments typically resolve with disorder remission, aligning with its brief duration and full recovery to premorbid status.	[3, 12]
Substance-Induced Psychosis (SIP)	Executive functioning, memory, attention.	Cognitive deficits mimic core psychotic disorders but vary based on substance type, usage duration/intensity, cessation patterns, and brain damage extent.	[44]

Table 1.
An overview of cognitive impairments in psychotic disorders.

the posterior subiculum, has emerged as a focal point in psychosis research. Lesions or dysfunctions in this region are linked to prominent symptoms like delusions and hallucinations. Connectivity patterns involving the posterior subiculum suggest that disruptions in this circuit contribute to the pathophysiology of psychosis [51, 52].

Furthermore, the prefrontal cortex (PFC), which governs higher cognitive processes, has been extensively studied in PSDs. Abnormalities in the PFC, particularly the dorsolateral region, are strongly associated with cognitive deficits observed in psychotic disorders [53, 54]. Reduced metabolic activity and cortical thinning in this region are well-documented findings. Although findings are conflicted in terms of whole brain matter volumes [55] more consistent results emerge when focusing specifically on gray matter [56, 57]. Furthermore, some studies have found smaller left prefrontal gray matter volumes among first-episode patients with schizophrenia compared with first-episode patients with affective psychosis and normal control subjects [58].

While the literature presents conflicting findings on connectivity patterns, recent studies have emphasized that connectivity between two key nodes of the default mode network, namely the precuneus-posterior cingulate cortex and the anterior cingulate cortex-medial prefrontal cortex, is heightened in response to ecological stimuli when compared to controls [53]. The PFC's connections to circuits implicated in psychosis make it a potential target for therapeutic interventions like transcranial magnetic stimulation (TMS).

Finally, the temporal lobes, including the superior temporal gyrus and parahippocampal gyrus, exhibit significant volume reductions in individuals with psychotic disorders. These changes are linked to impairments in memory, auditory processing, and social cognition, which are common in schizophrenia and related conditions [59].

3.2 Role of neurotransmitters (e.g., dopamine, glutamate)

The role of dopamine in schizophrenia has been a central focus of research, particularly in the context of the dopamine hypothesis. This theory suggests that hyperactivity within the mesolimbic dopamine pathway contributes to positive symptoms of schizophrenia, such as delusions and hallucinations. Dysregulation in this pathway affects the salience attribution process, leading to distorted perceptions and experiences [59, 60].

In addition to dopamine, glutamate has emerged as a critical neurotransmitter in understanding schizophrenia. Reduced function of the N-methyl D-aspartate (NMDA) receptor, a glutamate receptor subtype, has been consistently linked to the disorder. Postmortem studies reveal abnormally low levels of glutamate receptors in the brains of individuals with schizophrenia, suggesting that deficits in glutamatergic signaling may underlie cognitive and negative symptoms [61, 62]. This dysfunction highlights the interplay between neurotransmitter systems in the pathophysiology of schizophrenia, offering insights into potential therapeutic targets.

4. Neuropsychological assessment in psychosis

The previous sections have detailed the neuropsychological deficits and characteristics associated with psychotic disorders. In this regard, neuropsychological assessment serves as the critical first step in understanding the challenges and difficulties a person faces. It also provides valuable insights for personalizing and designing appropriate interventions tailored to their specific needs [11, 63].

The goal of neuropsychological assessment in psychosis is to understand the extent and nature of cognitive deficits, including impairments in attention, memory, executive function, and social cognition. Secondly, it aims to define personalized treatment approaches considering the intricate interactions among genetic, environmental, and psychological factors while also monitoring changes in cognitive function over time. Ultimately, the goal is to enhance daily functioning and improve overall quality of life [11].

The evaluation of important cognitive domains that are commonly impacted in people with PSD forms the basis of the neuropsychological screening tools employed in psychosis. These domains mainly include social cognition, memory and learning, and executive skills. Although a wide range of instruments have been reported in previous literature, the most commonly used instruments include the Trail Making Test, which evaluates processing speed, visual attention, task-switching, and cognitive flexibility [64, 65]. Another frequently used instrument is the Stroop Color and Word Test measuring processing speed and executive control processes, such as inhibition [66, 67]. Tasks assessing verbal learning and memory, such as the Rey Auditory Verbal Learning Test and the California Verbal Learning Test, are also frequently employed [68].

Furthermore, many studies utilize the MATRICS battery (Measurement and Treatment Research to Improve Cognition in Schizophrenia) [69], a standardized tool designed to assess domains frequently impaired in schizophrenia, including information processing speed, attention, vigilance, working memory, verbal learning, visual learning, reasoning, problem-solving, and social cognition. Additionally, global measures of intelligence and cognitive quotient, such as the Wechsler Adult Intelligence Scale, are often incorporated in the testing battery [70]. Moreover, depending on clinical requests or preferences, tests are also used to assess social skills and aspects of social cognition including emotion recognition tasks and theory of mind tasks [71, 72]. Finally, everyday life capacity, skills, and functioning are evaluated, as these are the most critical goals, having a direct impact on the individual's daily life and overall well-being. Instruments to assess everyday life activities frequently include question-based assessments such as the measures developed by Katz and colleagues [73] and Lawton and Brody [74].

5. Cognitive and functional correlates of psychosis

As outlined in previous sections, psychosis can manifest clinically in various schizotypal disorders, including schizophrenia, schizophreniform disorder, brief psychotic disorder, schizoaffective disorder, delusional disorder, as well as other specified schizophrenia spectrum and unspecified psychotic disorders according to the DSM-V [3]. Additionally, psychosis can co-occur with several mental health conditions such as bipolar disorder and severe depression, and neurological disorders such as Alzheimer's disease, Huntington's disease, Parkinson's disease, multiple sclerosis, and temporal lobe epilepsy [75–78]. Furthermore, factors such as brain tumors, strokes, infections, and substance abuse can precipitate or exacerbate psychotic episodes.

In all these instances, psychosis is accompanied by distinct neuropsychological impairments which affect individuals' cognitive and functional abilities. Research has highlighted that individuals with PSDs often exhibit deficits in cognitive domains such as memory (working and episodic memory), attention, executive skills, language, social cognition, and emotional regulation [12, 79]. These deficits are negatively associated with the ability to execute everyday life facets including employment, relationships, parenthood, and self-care, and are linked to dysfunction in the prefrontal cortex and particularly the dorsolateral region [12].

Additionally, these impairments can exacerbate the overall severity of psychotic symptoms and hinder recovery efforts. Hence, it is imperative to further explore how neurobiological and neuropsychological factors influence the daily functioning of individuals with PSDs. This information is particularly important for clinicians and professionals in order to plan and implement interventions to support individuals with PSD in daily functioning, including social interactions, employment, relationships, independence, self-care, and overall quality of life.

5.1 Employment

Employment rates among individuals with psychosis are generally low, though they vary depending on the phase of the illness. For those experiencing first-episode psychosis, employment rates range between 13% and 65% while for individuals with chronic schizophrenia, the rates are lower, typically ranging from 10 to 20% [25]. Interestingly, while psychotic symptoms are often characterized by prominent positive symptoms such as hallucinations, delusions, disorganized thoughts, and abnormal motor behaviors, as well as negative symptoms like affective flattening, alogia, avolition, and anhedonia, research suggests that neurocognition has the strongest impact on work behavior in patients with schizophrenia. Negative symptoms have a moderate effect, while positive symptoms appear to have only a peripheral influence [80]. These findings have been replicated in previous studies, highlighting the potential of psychosocial and neuropsychological interventions to alleviate daily functioning impairments among individuals with PSD.

5.2 Relationships and family

Relationships, family dynamics, and parenting are heavily impacted by the positive and negative symptoms of PSDs, as these often limit an individual's ability to consistently and appropriately meet the needs of their partner, children, or social circle. However, neuropsychological deficits also seem to play a central role in this regard.

Individuals with PSD frequently face communication and language difficulties. These may manifest as limited vocabulary, reduced fluency, poor pragmatic communication, and disorganized speech patterns [81, 82]. Impaired communication can lead to misunderstandings and frustration during family interactions, straining relationships. Furthermore, executive functioning deficits, which often present to people with PSD, can lead to difficulties with planning and organizing, and also hoarding tendencies [83, 84], making it challenging for them to contribute effectively to household responsibilities. These impairments may also affect emotional regulation, often resulting in an unstable environment, inconsistent parenting practices, and fluctuating partner or parental availability, all of which are critical for healthy relationships and effective child-rearing [85].

Finally, beyond their close relationships, individuals with PSD often face deficits in social cognition and theory of mind, frequently leading to social isolation and a limited social circle [86]. These challenges are further compounded by memory and processing speed issues, which make it difficult for them to participate in fast-paced conversations, understand humor, or feel comfortable joking with peers, often making them seem unempathetic or socially withdrawn [87]. These findings highlight the imperative of addressing these neuropsychological challenges to support individuals with PSD and their families.

5.3 Independence and financial management

Although not extensively researched, independence and financial management are frequently compromised in individuals with psychosis due to the multifaceted cognitive deficits and symptoms associated with the disorder. For example, impaired executive functioning, such as difficulties with planning, organization, and problem-solving, can make managing finances, paying bills, or budgeting particularly challenging [87, 88]. Additionally, poor decision-making skills and disorganized thinking may further complicate interactions with financial institutions, leading to missed payments or increased debt. These financial struggles often hinder overall independence, as individuals may become reliant on family members or caregivers for support [89].

These findings indicate that the daily challenges faced by individuals with psychotic disorders are largely driven by neuropsychological deficits. This underscores the potential benefits of psychosocial therapy, neuropsychological remediation, and cognitive enhancement as promising interventions in this field [90].

6. Neuropsychological deficits: Implications for treatment

As discussed in the previous sections, neuropsychological deficits in psychosis significantly impact functional outcomes and quality of life. In this context, various treatment options are available and emerging, mainly including psychopharmacological interventions, cognitive remediation therapies, psychosocial interventions, and neurostimulation.

6.1 Pharmacological therapies

The primary medication category utilized for the treatment of individuals with PSD is antipsychotic medications. Antipsychotic medications act as dopamine D1, D2, and D3 receptor antagonists, to address positive symptoms such as hallucinations and delusions [91, 92]. Yet, there is limited evidence regarding their impact on cognitive deficits while previous studies in animal models have even documented adverse effects on higher cognitive functions [93].

Second-generation antipsychotics have shown slight benefits in cognitive functioning compared to first-generation drugs, but overall effects remain modest [94]. Recent studies have explored adjunctive pharmacotherapies including antidepressants, antipsychotics, and cholinergic agents, targeting the acetylcholinergic, glutamatergic, and serotonergic systems. These approaches seem more favorable treatment options for individuals' cognitive profiles although findings require further validation [95–97].

6.2 Neuropsychological remediation therapy

Evidence supports the effectiveness of Cognitive Remediation/Neuropsychological Rehabilitation Therapy (CRT/NRT) in improving both cognitive performance and functional outcomes in individuals with PSD. CRT/NRT involves the completion of paper and pencil and/or digital/computer-based tasks targeting different cognitive functions with gradually increasing complexity [98]. The teaching of compensatory methods and techniques to make up for cognitive impairments is another aspect of CRT/NRT approaches [99].

A previous study by Lecardeur and colleagues revealed significant positive effects on mental flexibility and clinical symptoms in patients with PSD, following a novel CRT approach targeting mental flexibility in various scenarios closely aligned with everyday life situations [100]. Similarly, researchers have found CRT/NRT benefits on functional capacity in people with schizophrenia and also, planning and problem-solving skills [101] Furthermore, a recent study by McGurk and colleagues [102] demonstrated that CRT/NRT improved several cognitive measures, including executive skills, with no significant difference in outcomes whether CRT/NRT was used alone or combined with exercise.

Although CRT/NRT holds promise for the mitigation of cognitive deficits among individuals with PSD, research shows that patient engagement is affected by their positive symptoms (hallucinations, delusions) and negative symptoms (alogia, avolition), thus rendering the approach inconsistent in findings [103]. An overview of the most important findings on this topic can be found in **Table 2**.

6.3 Psychosocial interventions

Psychosocial interventions are key in supporting persons with PSD and enhancing outcomes like daily functioning and the control of both positive and negative symptoms. Cognitive Behavioral Therapy (CBT) is frequently used to help individuals manage symptoms by addressing maladaptive thoughts and behaviors [107, 108]. Through the development of coping mechanisms and the reduction of stress, cognitive functioning can be indirectly supported as well, and these people's self-efficacy and motivation can be increased [109].

Neuropsychological research highlights various cognitive impairments commonly observed in psychosis, such as deficits in attention, memory, and executive function. CBT can both influence and be influenced by these difficulties [11, 109]. For example, a person's capacity to recall and use schema-challenging strategies may be adversely affected by a short memory span or poor executive functioning. Thus, integrating neuropsychological insights can further improve CBT for psychosis. For instance, neuropsychological insights can improve the psychoeducational aspects of CBT by giving patients a better knowledge of the relationship between cognitive processes and symptoms and how these affect their everyday lives. Furthermore, executive difficulties are prominent among individuals with PSD, it can be very helpful to integrate techniques for enhancing planning, organizing, and problem-solving abilities into cognitive behavioral therapy. Activity scheduling, for instance, can assist patients better organize their daily routines and enhance their general functioning. Similarly, a strategy called graded exposure can improve executive functioning by exposing patients to frightening events progressively as they develop coping mechanisms.

6.4 Skills training

The everyday life challenges faced by individuals with PSD can be effectively addressed through skills training programs that focus on maintaining and developing practical abilities essential for daily living and social interactions. These programs,

Study	Sample	Intervention	Cognitive domains targeted	Outcome	Reference
Lecardeur et al., 2009	24 individuals with SCZ	Novel CRT approach targeting mental flexibility in everyday scenarios (2 interventions- 1 control group)	Mental state attribution and mental flexibility	Reduced clinical symptoms and cognitive complaints	[100]
Rodewald et al., 2011	89 people with SCZ	Computer-based planning and problem-solving or basic cognition training for 10, 45′ sessions	Planning, problem-solving and functionality	Positive effects on planning, problem-solving and functional capacity.	[101]
Hargreaves et al., 2015	56 individuals with psychosis	Web-based training for 8 weeks (control/ intervention)	Auditory and visual working memory	Positive effects on working memory performance	[104]
Vidarsdottir et al., 2019	49 people with a primary psychotic disorder	Group-based integrative cognitive remediation for 12 weeks (control/ intervention)	Several cognitive domains and social cognition	Positive effects on verbal memory, cognitive flexibility, working memory and theory of mind	[105]
McGurk et al., 2021	34 people with SCZ or bipolar disorder	CRT for 10 weeks (30 hours) or CRT with exercise (50-min sessions, 3 days/ week for 10 weeks)	Attention, working memory, verbal and visual learning, planning, executive function and clinical symptoms	Positive effects for both groups on most cognitive domains, no differential effect of exercise augmentation of CRT	[102]
Haugen et al., 2022	81 individuals with PSDs	Goal Management Training for 5 weeks (control/ intervention)	Executive function, daily function, clinical symptoms	Positive effects on self-reported executive functioning, everyday functionality, clinical symptoms, and neuropsychological performance	[106]

Table 2.
Key studies and outcomes of CRT/NRT in psychosis.

which aim to enhance living skills and social interactions for individuals with psychosis, often include vocational training and social skills development, both of which are vital for improving overall functioning and quality of life. Many of these programs utilize CRT/NRT techniques and primarily target adolescents and young adults due to the critical developmental period and the potential for positive outcomes within these population groups. For instance, a study by Uealand and Rund [110] on adolescents with early-onset psychosis demonstrated improvements not only in various cognitive measures, such as attention and executive skills but also in psychosocial functioning. Similarly, Eack and colleagues found that enhancements in social cognition among individuals with PSD following a CRT/NRT protocol significantly mediated indirect beneficial effects on employment status [111].

6.5 Neurostimulation therapies

Finally, neurostimulation therapies like transcranial magnetic stimulation (TMS) and Electroconvulsive Therapy (ECT) have been explored in treating cognitive deficits in PSDs. TMS is a non-invasive procedure that uses magnetic fields to stimulate nerve cells in the brain. Research suggests that TMS may improve cognitive functions, such as short-term memory, in people with schizophrenia by modulating neural activity associated with cognitive processes [112, 113]. On the other hand, ECT has been traditionally used for severe depression but is also being explored for its potential benefits in treating psychotic symptoms and associated cognitive deficits. While its primary use is not focused on cognition, some studies indicate that ECT protocols may lead to improvements in cognitive domains including information processing speed, attention, and visual learning, and even have lasting effects [114, 115].

According to previous studies, people with PSD perceive their cognitive deficits as a major culprit of their daily struggles, apart from the psycho-behavioral symptoms of psychosis itself [116]. This implies that people with psychosis view cognitive challenges as a significant obstacle to functioning. Therefore, it is encouraging that there are existing approaches, as well as combinations of these, that show promise in alleviating cognitive symptoms.

7. Emerging trends and future directions

The neuropsychological dimension of psychosis is accumulating increasing research interest due to its significant impact on daily functioning and quality of life. Emerging trends in treating neuropsychological deficiencies in psychosis focus on novel approaches, such as VR-based cognitive training, biomarker discovery, and personalized therapy [117, 118].

Through the simulation of real-life scenarios, virtual reality technology is becoming a powerful tool for training social, cognitive, and occupational skills among people with PSD. Although research is still limited in this field, VR shows promise as an adjective treatment in cognitive deficits, for example, executive skills, social difficulties (e.g., social cognition), and also work-related behaviors (e.g. behaviors needed for job interviews) [119, 120].

Additionally, a wide variety of indications, including peripheral, electrophysiological, neuroimaging, and neuropathological markers, have been examined in research on biomarkers for psychotic illnesses. No one biomarker was shown to be a reliable predictor in a big study that included 1478 biomarkers from 392,210 people. Nonetheless, a number of categories were found to have suggestive evidence, including biological markers like brain-derived neurotrophic factor, elevated transglutaminase autoantibody levels, and folate; electrophysiological markers like P50 sensory gating (P50 S2/S1 ratio), physical markers, neuroimaging markers, and physiological markers like high-frequency heart rate variability [118].

Last but not least, modern studies challenge the one-size-fits-all approach of previous years. Researchers specifically emphasize the need for tailored and individualized treatment plans because not all PSD patients respond equally to the same treatment protocol. Recent studies highlight the need for precision psychological, neuropsychological, and pharmaceutical treatments based on individual characteristics, factors, and biological profiles [121].

8. Challenges and limitations

Although neuropsychology is a promising field for the assessment and treatment of individuals with PSD, there are certain challenges and limitations when incorporating neuropsychology into therapeutic practice. These difficulties fall into three primary categories: integration problems, socioeconomic and cultural aspects, and ethical dilemmas.

Multidisciplinary cooperation, extra training, resources, and a common theoretical framework are needed to integrate neuropsychology into a comprehensive evaluation and treatment approach, which are not readily available in modern healthcare settings [122, 123]. Furthermore, in many countries, particularly those in Southern-Eastern Europe, information and awareness regarding the effects and benefits of neuropsychology are not widely known, which further exacerbates its underutilization in clinical practice. Moreover, research shows that socioeconomic and cultural factors directly impact neuropsychological testing and interventions. However, adaptations of neuropsychological tools are often nonrepresentative of specific countries, cultures, and languages, creating barriers that prevent their use [124]. Lastly, neuropsychological testing and interventions are, in many contexts, not covered by insurance or government programs. This lack of coverage makes them costly, particularly when they must be paid for out of pocket [123].

Lastly, conducting neuropsychological evaluations for people with PSD requires following ethical guidelines. The process and its ramifications must be completely understood by the individual, which can be especially difficult for people with cognitive disabilities. However, as the European Commission agenda emphasizes, a major ethical concern is the patient's right to access multidisciplinary teams, high-quality treatments, and health equity. This fact highlights that, in spite of the challenges, neuropsychological evaluation, therapy, and resources ought to be a part of contemporary clinical and medical environments.

9. Conclusion

In summary, research findings indicate that cognitive impairments are a major factor impacting everyday independence, functionality, and employment among people with PSDs. In this regard, neuropsychology is an essential field for comprehending and treating psychosis. Individuals with PSDs often find cognitive limitations to be the most upsetting aspect of their condition, in contrast to positive and negative symptoms, which tend to dominate clinical focus. These deficiencies impede important facets of daily life, hence underscoring the pressing need for focused and interdisciplinary interventions.

In this sense, multidisciplinary approaches have a key role in tackling PSD complexity in modern healthcare settings. The entire treatment of cognitive, emotional, and functional characteristics should be addressed through the collaboration of neuropsychologists, psychiatrists, neurologists, occupational therapists, and other experts.

Furthermore, treatment options that show promise in this field include neuropsychological therapies like CRT/NRT. To fully understand their effects and evaluate how these interventions improve daily functioning and quality of life, further studies are needed. Future studies should focus on exploring the impact of personalized CRT/NRT protocols, the generalizability of the effects in daily life tasks, as well as the development and testing of culturally sensitive instruments and standards.

Author details

Sotiria Moza[1,2]* and Savvina Chrysostomou[1]

1 Noesis Cognitive Center and Tech Solutions Ltd, Nicosia, Cyprus

2 Lab of Cognitive Neuroscience, School of Psychology Aristotle University of Thessaloniki, Thessaloniki, Greece

*Address all correspondence to: sotiria@noesis.cy

References

[1] Schizophrenia [Internet]. [cited 2024 Dec 10]. Available from: https://www.who.int/news-room/fact-sheets/detail/schizophrenia?utm_source=chatgpt.com

[2] Moreno-Küstner B, Martín C, Pastor L. Prevalence of psychotic disorders and its association with methodological issues. A systematic review and meta-analyses. PLoS One [Internet]. 2018;**13**(4):e0195687. DOI: 10.1371/journal.pone.0195687

[3] American Psychiatric Association. Diagnostic and Statistical Manual of Mental Disorders (DSM-5) [Internet]. American Psychiatric Publishing; 2021. Available from: https://books.google.com/books/about/Diagnostic_and_Statistical_Manual_of_Men.html?hl=&id=_8KtzgEACAAJ

[4] Heckers S, Barch DM, Bustillo J, Gaebel W, Gur R, Malaspina D, et al. Structure of the psychotic disorders classification in DSM-5. Schizophrenia research. [Internet] 2016;**150**(1):11-14. 2016. [cited 2024 Dec 22]. DOI: 10.1176/appi.focus.140307

[5] Alkan E, Davies G, Evans SL. Cognitive impairment in schizophrenia: Relationships with cortical thickness in fronto-temporal regions, and dissociability from symptom severity. npj Schizophrenia [Internet]. 2021;7(1):1-9. [cited 2024 Dec 22]. Available from: https://www.nature.com/articles/s41537-021-00149-0

[6] Ragland JD, Yoon J, Minzenberg MJ, Carter CS. Neuroimaging of cognitive disability in schizophrenia: Search for a pathophysiological mechanism. International Review of Psychiatry (Abingdon, England) [Internet]. 2007;**19**(4):417. [cited 2024 Dec 22]. Available from: https://pmc.ncbi.nlm.nih.gov/articles/PMC4332575/

[7] Khalil M, Hollander P, Raucher-Chéné D, Lepage M, Lavigne KM. Structural brain correlates of cognitive function in schizophrenia: A meta-analysis. Neuroscience & Biobehavioral Reviews. 2022;**132**:37-49. DOI: 10.1016/j.neubiorev.2021.11.034

[8] Martini F, Spangaro M, Bechi M, Agostoni G, Buonocore M, Sapienza J, et al. Improving outcome of treatment-resistant schizophrenia: Effects of cognitive remediation therapy. European Archives of Psychiatry and Clinical Neuroscience [Internet]. 2023;**274**(6):1473-1481. [cited 2024 Dec 22]. DOI: 10.1007/s00406-023-01731-6

[9] Harris N, Williams S, Bradshaw T. Psychosocial Interventions for People with Schizophrenia: A Practical Guide for Mental Health Workers [Internet]. Bloomsbury Publishing; 2017. 286 p. Available from: https://books.google.com/books/about/Psychosocial_Interventions_for_People_wi.html?hl=&id=EhpHEAAAQBAJ

[10] National Institute of Mental Health. Understanding Psychosis. U.S. Department of Health and Human Services. 2024. Available from: https://infocenter.nimh.nih.gov/publications/understanding-psychosis [Accessed: December 8, 2024]

[11] Gkintoni E, Skokou M, Gourzis P. Integrating clinical neuropsychology and psychotic spectrum disorders: A systematic analysis of cognitive dynamics, interventions, and underlying mechanisms. Medicina [Internet]. 2024;**60**(4):645. [cited 2024 Dec 10].

Available from: https://www.mdpi.com/1648-9144/60/4/645

[12] Sheffield JM, Karcher NR, Barch DM. Cognitive deficits in psychotic disorders: A lifespan perspective. Neuropsychology Review [Internet]. 2018;**28**(4):509-533. DOI: 10.1007/s11065-018-9388-2

[13] van Os J, Linscott RJ, Myin-Germeys I, Delespaul P, Krabbendam L. A systematic review and meta-analysis of the psychosis continuum: Evidence for a psychosis proneness-persistence-impairment model of psychotic disorder. Psychological Medicine [Internet]. 2009;**39**(2):179-195. DOI: 10.1017/S0033291708003814

[14] American Psychiatric Association DS, American Psychiatric Association DS. Diagnostic and statistical manual of mental disorders: DSM-5. Washington, DC: American psychiatric association; 2013. DOI: 10.1176/appi.books.9780890425596

[15] Arciniegas DB. Psychosis. Continuum (Minneap Minn) [Internet]. 2015;**21**(3 Behavioral Neurology and Neuropsychiatry):715-736. DOI: 10.1212/01.CON.0000466662.89908.e7

[16] Tandon R, Nasrallah HA, Keshavan MS. Schizophrenia, "just the facts" 4. Clinical features and conceptualization. Schizophrenia Research [Internet]. 2009;**110**(1-3):1-23. DOI: 10.1016/j.schres.2009.03.005

[17] American Psychiatric Association. Cautionary statement for forensic use of DSM-5. In: Diagnostic and Statistical Manual of Mental Disorders. 5th ed. 2013. DOI: 10.1176/appi.books.9780890425596.CautionaryStatement

[18] World Health Organization. World Health Statistics. Monitoring health for the Sdgs. Sustainable Development Goals [Internet]. 2019;**2019**. 126 p. Available from: https://books.google.com/books/about/World_Health_Statistics_2019.html?hl=&id=C9oizQEACAAJ

[19] Howes OD, Kapur S. The dopamine hypothesis of schizophrenia: Version III--The final common pathway. Schizophrenia Bulletin [Internet]. 2009;**35**(3):549-562. DOI: 10.1093/schbul/sbp006

[20] Li M, Spaulding WD. The Neuropsychopathology of Schizophrenia: Molecules, Brain Systems, Motivation, and Cognition [Internet]. Springer; 2016. 264 p. Available from: https://books.google.com/books/about/The_Neuropsychopathology_of_Schizophreni.html?hl=&id=MoxFDAAAQBAJ

[21] Heinrichs RW, Zakzanis KK. Neurocognitive deficit in schizophrenia: A quantitative review of the evidence. Neuropsychology [Internet]. 1998;**12**(3):426-445. DOI: 10.1037//0894-4105.12.3.426

[22] Bilder RM, Goldman RS, Robinson D, Reiter G, Bell L, Bates JA, et al. Neuropsychology of first-episode schizophrenia: Initial characterization and clinical correlates. American Journal of Psychiatry [Internet]. 2000;**157**(4):549-559. DOI: 10.1176/appi.ajp.157.4.549

[23] Ventura J, Hellemann GS, Thames AD, Koellner V, Nuechterlein KH. Symptoms as mediators of the relationship between neurocognition and functional outcome in schizophrenia: A meta-analysis. Schizophrenian Research [Internet]. 2009;**113**(2-3):189-199. DOI: 10.1016/j.schres.2009.03.035

[24] Fett AKJ, Viechtbauer W, Dominguez M d G, Penn DL, van Os J,

Krabbendam L. The relationship between neurocognition and social cognition with functional outcomes in schizophrenia: A meta-analysis. Neuroscience & Biobehavioral Review [Internet]. 2011;**35**(3):573-588. DOI: 10.1016/j.neubiorev.2010.07.001

[25] Marwaha S, Johnson S. Schizophrenia and employment - a review. Social Psychiatry and Psychiatric Epidemiology [Internet]. 2004;**39**(5):337-349. DOI: 10.1007/s00127-004-0762-4

[26] Tan BL. Profile of cognitive problems in schizophrenia and implications for vocational functioning. Australian Occupational Therapy Journal [Internet]. 2009;**56**(4):220-228. [cited 2024 Dec 10]. DOI: 10.1111/j.1440-1630.2008.00759.x

[27] Becker HE, Nieman DH, Dingemans PM, van de Fliert JR, De Haan L, Linszen DH. Verbal fluency as a possible predictor for psychosis. European Psychiatry [Internet]. 2010;**25**(2):105-110. [cited 2024 Dec 10]. Available from: https://www.cambridge.org/core/services/aop-cambridge-core/content/view/FBC61A9A92FFDF2DE024DF62A99B68AC/S0924933800066165a.pdf/div-class-title-verbal-fluency-as-a-possible-predictor-for-psychosis-div.pdf

[28] Website [Internet]. Available from: https://karger.com/psp/article-abstract/46/4/241/294301

[29] Leanza L, Egloff L, Studerus E, Andreou C, Heitz U, Ittig S, Beck K, Uttinger M, Riecher-Rössler A. The relationship between negative symptoms and cognitive functioning in patients at clinical high risk for psychosis. Psychiatry research. 1 Oct 2018;**268**:21-27. [cited 2024 Dec 10]. DOI: 10.1016/j.psychres.2018.06.047

[30] Faerden A, Vaskinn A, Finset A, Agartz I, Ann Barrett E, Friis S, et al. Apathy is associated with executive functioning in first episode psychosis. BMC Psychiatry [Internet]. 2009;**9**(1):1-8. [cited 2024 Dec 10]. DOI: 10.1186/1471-244X-9-1

[31] De la Serna E, Puig O, Mezquida G, Moreno-Izco L, Merchan-Naranjo J, Amoretti S, et al. Relationship between cognition and age at onset of first-episode psychosis: Comparative study between adolescents, young adults, and adults. Eur Child Adolesc Psychiatry [Internet]. 2023;**32**(4):639-649. DOI: 10.1007/s00787-021-01901-8

[32] Pedruzo B, Aymerich C, Pacho M, Herrero J, Laborda M, Bordenave M, et al. Longitudinal change in neurocognitive functioning in children and adolescents at clinical high risk for psychosis: A systematic review. European Child & Adolescent Psychiatry [Internet]. 2024;**33**(10):3377-3387. DOI: 10.1007/s00787-023-02221-9

[33] Carey E, Gillan D, Healy C, Dooley N, Campbell D, McGrane J, et al. Early adult mental health, functional and neuropsychological outcomes of young people who have reported psychotic experiences: A 10-year longitudinal study. Psychological Medicine [Internet]. 2021;**51**(11):1861-1869. DOI: 10.1017/S0033291720000616

[34] Vermeulen T, Lauwers T, Van Diermen L, Sabbe BG, van der Mast RC, Giltay EJ. Cognitive deficits in older adults with psychotic depression: a meta-analysis. The American Journal of Geriatric Psychiatry. 1 Dec 2019;**27**(12):1334-1344. [cited 2024 Dec 10]. DOI: 10.1016/j.jagp.2019.07.011

[35] Ismail Z, Ghahremani M, Amlish Munir M, Fischer CE, Smith EE, Creese B. A longitudinal study of late-life

psychosis and incident dementia and the potential effects of race and cognition. Nature Mental Health [Internet]. 2023;**1**(4):273-283. [cited 2024 Dec 10]. Available from: https://www.nature.com/articles/s44220-023-00043-x

[36] Dickinson D, Ramsey ME, Gold JM. Overlooking the obvious: A meta-analytic comparison of digit symbol coding tasks and other cognitive measures in schizophrenia. Archives of General Psychiatry [Internet]. 2007;**64**(5):532-542. DOI: 10.1001/archpsyc.64.5.532

[37] Seabury RD, Cannon TD. Memory impairments and psychosis prediction: A scoping review and theoretical overview. Neuropsychology Review [Internet]. 2020;**30**(4):521-545. DOI: 10.1007/s11065-020-09464-2

[38] Erlenmeyer-Kimling L, Rock D, Roberts SA, Janal M, Kestenbaum C, Cornblatt B, et al. Attention, memory, and motor skills as childhood predictors of schizophrenia-related psychoses: The New York high-risk project. American Journal of Psychiatry [Internet]. 2000;**157**(9):1416-1422. DOI: 10.1176/appi.ajp.157.9.1416

[39] Martin AK, Mowry B, Reutens D, Robinson GA. Executive functioning in schizophrenia: Unique and shared variance with measures of fluid intelligence. Brain and Cognition [Internet]. 2015;**99**:57-67. DOI: 10.1016/j.bandc.2015.07.009

[40] de Boer JN, van Hoogdalem M, Mandl RCW, Brummelman J, Voppel AE, Begemann MJH, et al. Language in schizophrenia: Relation with diagnosis, symptomatology and white matter tracts. NPJ Schizophrenia [Internet]. 2020;**6**(1):10. DOI: 10.1038/s41537-020-0099-3

[41] Watson AJ, Harrison L, Preti A, Wykes T, Cella M. Cognitive trajectories following onset of psychosis: A meta-analysis. British Journal of Psychiatry [Internet]. 2022;**221**(6):714-721. DOI: 10.1192/bjp.2022.131

[42] Mann-Wrobel MC,Carreno JT, Dickinson D. Meta-analysis of neuropsychological functioning in euthymic bipolar disorder: An update and investigation of moderator variables. Bipolar Disorders [Internet]. 2011;**13**(4):334-342. DOI: 10.1111/j.1399-5618.2011.00935.x

[43] Martínez-Arán A, Vieta E, Colom F, Reinares M, Benabarre A, Gastó C, et al. Cognitive dysfunctions in bipolar disorder: Evidence of neuropsychological disturbances. Psychotherapy and Psychosomatics [Internet]. 2000;**69**(1):2-18. DOI: 10.1159/000012361

[44] Gicas KM, Parmar PK, Fabiano GF, Mashhadi F. Substance-induced psychosis and cognitive functioning: A systematic review. Psychiatry Research [Internet]. 2022;**308**:114361. DOI: 10.1016/j.psychres.2021.114361

[45] Lizano P, Lutz O, Ling G, Lee AM, Eum S, Bishop JR, et al. Association of choroid plexus enlargement with cognitive, inflammatory, and structural phenotypes across the psychosis spectrum. American Journal of Psychiatry [Internet]. 2019;**176**(7):564-572. DOI: 10.1176/appi.ajp.2019.18070825

[46] Senay O, Seethaler M, Makris N, Yeterian E, Rushmore J, Cho KIK, et al. A preliminary choroid plexus volumetric study in individuals with psychosis. Human Brain Mapping [Internet]. 2023;**44**(6):2465-2478. DOI: 10.1002/hbm.26224

[47] Bannai D, Lutz O, Lizano P. Neuroimaging considerations when

investigating choroid plexus morphology in idiopathic psychosis. Schizophrenia Research [Internet]. 2020;**224**:19-21. DOI: 10.1016/j.schres.2020.07.013

[48] Zhang Y, Lu Z, Sun Y, Zhang X, Li Q, Li M, et al. Predictive role of pulvinar in social functional outcome of schizophrenia. Psychiatry Research [Internet]. 2023;**327**:115419. DOI: 10.1016/j.psychres.2023.115419

[49] Anticevic A, Halassa MM. The thalamus in psychosis spectrum disorder. Frontiers in Neuroscience [Internet]. 2023;**17**:1163600. DOI: 10.3389/fnins.2023.1163600

[50] Huang AS, Rogers BP, Sheffield JM, Jalbrzikowski ME, Anticevic A, Blackford JU, et al. Thalamic nuclei volumes in psychotic disorders and in youths with psychosis spectrum symptoms. American Journal of Psychiatry [Internet]. 2020;**177**(12):1159-1167. DOI: 10.1176/appi.ajp.2020.19101099

[51] Nakahara S, Matsumoto M, van Erp TGM. Hippocampal subregion abnormalities in schizophrenia: A systematic review of structural and physiological imaging studies. Neuropsychopharmacology Reports [Internet]. 2018;**38**(4):156-166. DOI: 10.1002/npr2.12031

[52] Cao P, Li Y, Dong Y, Tang Y, Xu G, Si Q, et al. Different structural connectivity patterns in the subregions of the thalamus, hippocampus, and cingulate cortex between schizophrenia and psychotic bipolar disorder. Journal of Affective Disorders [Internet]. 2024;**363**:269-281. DOI: 10.1016/j.jad.2024.07.077

[53] Rikandi E, Mäntylä T, Lindgren M, Kieseppä T, Suvisaari J, Raij TT. Connectivity of the precuneus-posterior cingulate cortex with the anterior cingulate cortex-medial prefrontal cortex differs consistently between control subjects and first-episode psychosis patients during a movie stimulus. Schizophrenia Research [Internet]. 2018;**199**:235-242. DOI: 10.1016/j.schres.2018.03.018

[54] Callicott JH, Bertolino A, Mattay VS, Langheim FJ, Duyn J, Coppola R, et al. Physiological dysfunction of the dorsolateral prefrontal cortex in schizophrenia revisited. Cerebral Cortex [Internet]. 2000;**10**(11):1078-1092. DOI: 10.1093/cercor/10.11.1078

[55] Shenton ME, Dickey CC, Frumin M, McCarley RW. A review of MRI findings in schizophrenia. Schizophrenia research. 15 Apr 2001;**49**(1-2):1-52. [cited 2024 Dec 10]. DOI: 10.1016/S0920-9964(01)00163-3

[56] Molina V, Sanz J, Sarramea F, Benito C, Palomo T. Lower prefrontal gray matter volume in schizophrenia in chronic but not in first episode schizophrenia patients. Psychiatry Research [Internet]. 2004;**131**(1):45-56. DOI: 10.1016/j.pscychresns.2004.01.005

[57] Website [Internet]. Available from: 10.1093/cercor/11.4.374

[58] Wiegand LC, Warfield SK, Levitt JJ, Hirayasu Y, Salisbury DF, Heckers S, et al. Prefrontal cortical thickness in first-episode psychosis: A magnetic resonance imaging study. Biological Psychiatry [Internet]. 2004;**55**(2):131-140. DOI: 10.1016/j.biopsych.2003.07.009

[59] Kaur A, Basavanagowda DM, Rathod B, Mishra N, Fuad S, Nosher S, et al. Structural and functional alterations of the temporal lobe in schizophrenia: A literature review.

Cureus [Internet]. 2020;**12**(10):e11177. DOI: 10.7759/cureus.11177

[60] Seidman LJ, Pantelis C, Keshavan MS, Faraone SV, Goldstein JM, Horton NJ, et al. A review and new report of medial temporal lobe dysfunction as a vulnerability indicator for schizophrenia: A magnetic resonance imaging morphometric family study of the parahippocampal gyrus. Schizophrenia Bulletin [Internet]. 2003;**29**(4):803-830. DOI: 10.1093/oxfordjournals.schbul.a007048

[61] Nakazawa K, Sapkota K. The origin of NMDA receptor hypofunction in schizophrenia. Pharmacology & therapeutics. 1 Jan 2020;**205**:107426. [cited 2024 Dec 10]. DOI: 10.1016/j.pharmthera.2019.107426

[62] Balu DT. The NMDA receptor and schizophrenia: from pathophysiology to treatment. Advances in pharmacology. Jan 1 2016;**76**:351-82. [cited 2024 Dec 10]. DOI: 10.1016/bs.apha.2016.01.006

[63] Cowman M, Lonergan E, Burke T, Bowie CR, Corvin A, Morris DW, et al. Evidence supporting the use of a brief cognitive assessment in routine clinical assessment for psychosis. Schizophrenia (Heidelb) [Internet]. 2022;**8**(1):113. DOI: 10.1038/s41537-022-00322-z

[64] Armitage SG. An Analysis of Certain Psychological Tests Used for the Evaluation of Brain Injury [Internet]. 1946. 346 p. Available from: https://books.google.com/books/about/An_Analysis_of_Certain_Psychological_Tes.html?hl=&id=dswSAAAAIAAJ

[65] Laere E, Tee SF, Tang PY. Assessment of cognition in schizophrenia using trail making test: A meta-analysis. Psychiatry Investigation [Internet]. 2018;**15**(10):945-955. DOI: 10.30773/pi.2018.07.22

[66] Website [Internet]. Available from: 10.1037/h0054651

[67] Laurenson C, Gorwood P, Orsat M, Lhuillier JP, Le Gall D, Richard-Devantoy S. Cognitive control and schizophrenia: The greatest reliability of the Stroop task. Psychiatry Research. 30 May 2015;**227**(1):10-6. [cited 2024 Dec 10]. DOI: 10.1016/j.psychres.2015.03.004

[68] Kilciksiz CM, Keefe R, Benoit J, Öngür D, Torous J. Verbal memory measurement towards digital perspectives in first-episode psychosis: A review. Schizophrenia Research Cognition [Internet]. 2020;**21**:100177. DOI: 10.1016/j.scog.2020.100177

[69] Hyman SE, Fenton WS, Medicine. What are the right targets for psychopharmacology? Science [Internet]. 2003;**299**(5605):350-351. DOI: 10.1126/science.1077141

[70] Michel NM, Goldberg JO, Heinrichs RW, Miles AA, Ammari N, McDermid VS. WAIS-IV profile of cognition in schizophrenia. Assessment [Internet]. 2013;**20**(4):462-473. DOI: 10.1177/1073191113478153

[71] Fantie BD, Kosmidis MH, Giannakou M, Moza S, Karavatos A, Bozikas VP. What is going on? The process of generating questions about emotion and social cognition in bipolar disorder and schizophrenia with cartoon situations and faces. Brain Sciences [Internet]. 2018;**8**(4):68. [cited 2024 Dec 10]. Available from: https://www.mdpi.com/2076-3425/8/4/68

[72] Barbato M, Liu L, Cadenhead KS, Cannon TD, Cornblatt BA, McGlashan TH, et al. Theory of mind, emotion recognition and social perception in individuals at clinical high risk for psychosis: Findings

from the NAPLS-2 cohort. Schizophrenia Research Cognition [Internet]. 2015;**2**(3):133-139. DOI: 10.1016/j.scog.2015.04.004

[73] Katz S, Ford AB, Moskowitz RW, Jackson BA, Jaffe MW. Studies of illness in the aged. The index of adl: A standardized measure of biological and psychosocial function. JAMA [Internet]. 1963;**185**:914-919. DOI: 10.1001/jama.1963.03060120024016

[74] Lawton MP, Brody EM. Assessment of older people: Self-maintaining and instrumental activities of daily living. Gerontologist [Internet]. 1969;**9**(3):179-186. Available from: https://www.ncbi.nlm.nih.gov/pubmed/5349366

[75] Imbimbo C, Cotta Ramusino M, Leone S, Mazzacane F, De Franco V, Gatti A, et al. Emerging pharmacological approaches for psychosis and agitation in Alzheimer's disease. CNS Drugs [Internet]. 2024:1-18. DOI: 10.1007/s40263-024-01133-9

[76] Angelopoulou E, Bougea A, Papageorgiou SG, Villa C. Psychosis in Parkinson's disease: A lesson from genetics. Genes. 20 Jun 2022;**13**(6):1099. DOI: 10.3390/ genes13061099

[77] Sone D. Neurobiological mechanisms of psychosis in epilepsy: Findings from neuroimaging studies. Frontiers in Psychiatry [Internet]. 2022;**13**:1079295. DOI: 10.3389/fpsyt.2022.1079295

[78] Romero-Luna G, Mejía-Pérez SI, Ramírez-Cruz J, Aguilar-Hidalgo KM, Ocampo-Díaz KM, Moscardini-Martelli J, et al. Schizophrenia-like psychosis presented in a patient with a temporal lobe tumor: A case report. Cureus [Internet]. 2022;**14**(9):e29034. DOI: 10.7759/cureus.29034

[79] Smucny J, Dienel SJ, Lewis DA, Carter CS. Mechanisms underlying dorsolateral prefrontal cortex contributions to cognitive dysfunction in schizophrenia. Neuropsychopharmacology [Internet]. 2022;**47**(1):292-308. DOI: 10.1038/s41386-021-01089-0

[80] Giordano GM, Pezzella P, Mucci A, Austin SF, Erfurth A, Glenthøj B, et al. Negative symptoms and social cognition as mediators of the relationship between neurocognition and functional outcome in schizophrenia. Frontiers in Psychiatry [Internet]. 2024;**15**:1333711. DOI: 10.3389/fpsyt.2024.1333711

[81] Gargano G, Caletti E, Perlini C, Turtulici N, Bellani M, Bonivento C, et al. Language production impairments in patients with a first episode of psychosis. PLoS One [Internet]. 2022;**17**(8):e0272873. DOI: 10.1371/journal.pone.0272873

[82] Ehlen F, Montag C, Leopold K, Heinz A. Linguistic findings in persons with schizophrenia-a review of the current literature. Frontiers in Psychology [Internet]. 2023;**14**:1287706. DOI: 10.3389/fpsyg.2023.1287706

[83] Schou ML, Urfer-Parnas A, Parnas J. The hoarding phenomenon in schizophrenia Spectrum disorders. Psychopathology [Internet]. 2020;**53**(2):111-118. DOI: 10.1159/000508453

[84] Heffernan T, Hamilton C, Neave N. Self-reported memory and executive function in adult non-clinical hoarders. Applied Neuropsychology Adult [Internet]. 2023;**30**(2):153-158. DOI: 10.1080/23279095.2021.1917578

[85] Ludwig L, Werner D, Lincoln TM. The relevance of cognitive emotion regulation to psychotic symptoms - a systematic review and meta-analysis. Clinical Psychology Review [Internet].

2019;**72**:101746. DOI: 10.1016/j.cpr.2019.101746

[86] van Neerven T, Bos DJ, van Haren NE. Deficiencies in theory of mind in patients with schizophrenia, bipolar disorder, and major depressive disorder: A systematic review of secondary literature. Neuroscience & Biobehavioral Reviews [Internet]. 2021;**120**:249-261. DOI: 10.1016/j.neubiorev.2020.11.011

[87] Volovik DD, Omelchenko MA, Ivanova AM. Emotional response to humour perception and gelotophobia among healthy individuals and patients with schizophrenia and depression, with signs of a high clinical risk of psychosis. Consort Psychiatrary [Internet]. 2021;**2**(1):8-17. DOI: 10.17816/CP65

[88] Twamley EW, Doshi RR, Nayak GV, Palmer BW, Golshan S, Heaton RK, et al. Generalized cognitive impairments, ability to perform everyday tasks, and level of independence in community living situations of older patients with psychosis. American Journal of Psychiatry [Internet]. 2002;**159**(12):2013-2020. DOI: 10.1176/appi.ajp.159.12.2013

[89] Foldemo A, Ek AC, Bogren L. Needs in outpatients with schizophrenia, assessed by the patients themselves and their parents and staff. Social Psychiatry and Psychiatric Epidemiology [Internet]. 2004;**39**(5):381-385. [cited 2024 Dec 10]. DOI: 10.1007/s00127-004-0750-8

[90] Fitapelli B, Lindenmayer JP. Advances in cognitive remediation training in schizophrenia: A review. Brain Sciences. 18 Jan 2022;**12**(2):129. DOI: 10.3390/brainsci12020129

[91] Németh G, Falkai P, Szulc A. Novel Antipsychotics Within and Beyond Clinical Trials: The Treatment of Overlapping Psychiatric Disorders with D3-D2 Partial Agonists [Internet]. Frontiers Media SA; 2022. 269 p. Available from: https://books.google.com/books/about/Novel_Antipsychotics_Within_and_Beyond_C.html?hl=&id=dSibEAAAQBAJ

[92] Davis JM, Casper R. Antipsychotic drugs: Clinical pharmacology and therapeutic use. Drugs [Internet]. 1977;**14**(4):260-282. DOI: 10.2165/00003495-197714040-00002

[93] Sawaguchi T, Goldman-Rakic PS. The role of D1-dopamine receptor in working memory: Local injections of dopamine antagonists into the prefrontal cortex of rhesus monkeys performing an oculomotor delayed-response task. Journal of Neurophysiology [Internet]. 1994;**71**(2):515-528. DOI: 10.1152/jn.1994.71.2.515

[94] Hill SK, Bishop JR, Palumbo D, Sweeney JA. Effect of second-generation antipsychotics on cognition: Current issues and future challenges. Expert Review of Neurotherapeutics [Internet]. 2010;**10**(1):43-57. DOI: 10.1586/ern.09.143

[95] Vita A, Nibbio G, Barlati S. Pharmacological treatment of cognitive impairment associated with schizophrenia: State of the art and future perspectives. Schizophrenia Bulletin Open [Internet]. 2024;**5**(1):sgae013. DOI: 10.1093/schizbullopen/sgae013

[96] Hsu WY, Lane HY, Lin CH. Medications used for cognitive enhancement in patients with schizophrenia, bipolar disorder, Alzheimer's disease, and Parkinson's disease. Frontiers in Psychiatry [Internet]. 2018;**9**:91. DOI: 10.3389/fpsyt.2018.00091

[97] Choi KH, Wykes T, Kurtz MM. Adjunctive pharmacotherapy for

cognitive deficits in schizophrenia: Meta-analytical investigation of efficacy. British Journal of Psychiatry [Internet]. 2013;**203**(3):172-178. DOI: 10.1192/bjp.bp.111.107359

[98] Medalia A, Choi J. Cognitive remediation in schizophrenia. Neuropsychology Review [Internet]. 2009;**19**(3):353-364. DOI: 10.1007/s11065-009-9097-y

[99] Allott K, van-der-El K, Bryce S, Parrish EM, SR MG, Hetrick S, et al. Compensatory interventions for cognitive impairments in psychosis: A systematic review and meta-analysis. Schizophrenia Bulletin [Internet]. 2020;**46**(4):869-883. DOI: 10.1093/schbul/sbz134

[100] Lecardeur L, Stip E, Giguere M, BlouinG,RodriguezJP,Champagne-LavauM. Effects of cognitive remediation therapies on psychotic symptoms and cognitive complaints in patients with schizophrenia and related disorders: A randomized study. Schizophrenia Research [Internet]. 2009;**111**(1-3):153-158. DOI: 10.1016/j.schres.2009.03.029

[101] Rodewald K, Rentrop M, Holt DV, Roesch-Ely D, Backenstrass M, Funke J, et al. Planning and problem-solving training for patients with schizophrenia: A randomized controlled trial. BMC Psychiatry [Internet]. 2011;**11**:73. DOI: 10.1186/1471-244X-11-73

[102] McGurk SR, Otto MW, Fulford D, Cutler Z, Mulcahy LP, Talluri SS, et al. A randomized controlled trial of exercise on augmenting the effects of cognitive remediation in persons with severe mental illness. Journal of Psychiatric Research. 1 Jul 2021;**139**:38-46. [cited 2024 Dec 22]. DOI: 10.1016/j.jpsychires.2021.04.033

[103] Altman RAE, Tan EJ, Rossell SL. Factors impacting access and engagement of cognitive remediation therapy for people with schizophrenia: A systematic review. Canadian Journal of Psychiatry [Internet]. 2023;**68**(3):139-151. DOI: 10.1177/07067437221129073

[104] Hargreaves A, Dillon R, Anderson-Schmidt H, Corvin A, Fitzmaurice B, Castorina M, Robertson IH, Donohoe G. Computerised working-memory focused cognitive remediation therapy for psychosis—A preliminary study. Schizophrenia Research. 1 Dec 2015;**169**(1-3):135-140. [cited 2024 Dec 22]. DOI: 10.1016/j.schres.2015.09.004

[105] Vidarsdottir OG, Roberts DL, Twamley EW, Gudmundsdottir B, Sigurdsson E, Magnusdottir BB. Integrative cognitive remediation for early psychosis: results from a randomized controlled trial. Psychiatry Research. 1 Mar 2019;**273**:690-698. [cited 2024 Dec 22]. DOI: 10.1016/j.psychres.2019.02.007

[106] Haugen I, Stubberud J, Haug E, McGurk SR, Hovik KT, Ueland T, et al. A randomized controlled trial of goal management training for executive functioning in schizophrenia spectrum disorders or psychosis risk syndromes. BMC Psychiatry [Internet]. 2022;**22**(1):1-17. [cited 2024 Dec 22]. DOI: 10.1186/s12888-022-04197-3

[107] Hayward M, Berry K, Bremner S, Cavanagh K, Dodgson G, Fowler D, et al. Increasing access to CBT for psychosis patients: Study protocol for a randomised controlled trial evaluating brief, targeted CBT for distressing voices delivered by assistant psychologists (GiVE3). Trials [Internet]. 2023;**24**(1):588. DOI: 10.1186/s13063-023-07611-7

[108] Hagen R, Turkington D, Berge T, Gråwe RW. CBT for Psychosis: A Symptom-Based Approach [Internet].

Routledge; 2013. 291 p. Available from: https://books.google.com/books/about/CBT_for_Psychosis.html?hl=&id=D_ZbpcBVXY8C

[109] Reddy LF, Glynn SM, McGovern JE, Sugar CA, Reavis EA, Green MF. A novel psychosocial intervention for motivational negative symptoms in schizophrenia: Combined motivational interviewing and CBT. American Journal of Psychiatry [Internet]. 2023;**180**(5):367-376. DOI: 10.1176/appi.ajp.20220243

[110] Ueland T, Rund BR. Cognitive remediation for adolescents with early onset psychosis: A 1-year follow-up study. Acta Psychiatrica Scandinavica [Internet]. 2005;**111**(3):193-201. DOI: 10.1111/j.1600-0447.2004.00503.x

[111] Roberts DL, Penn DL. Social Cognition in Schizophrenia: From Evidence to Treatment [Internet]. USA: Oxford University Press; 2013. 449 p. Available from: https://books.google.com/books/about/Social_Cognition_in_Schizophrenia.html?hl=&id=Cnz8jLKzpHkC

[112] Mao J, Fan K, Zhang Y, Wen N, Fang X, Ye X, et al. 10 Hz repetitive transcranial magnetic stimulation (rTMS) may improve cognitive function: An exploratory study of schizophrenia patients with auditory hallucinations. Heliyon [Internet]. 2023;**9**(9):e19912. DOI: 10.1016/j.heliyon.2023.e19912

[113] Li X, Dai J, Liu Q, Zhao Z, Zhang X. Efficacy and safety of non-invasive brain stimulation on cognitive function for cognitive impairment associated with schizophrenia: A systematic review and meta-analysis. Journal of Psychiatric Research [Internet]. 2024;**170**:174-186. DOI: 10.1016/j.jpsychires.2023.12.003

[114] Mohn C, Rund BR. Maintained improvement of neurocognitive function in major depressive disorders 6 months after ECT. Frontiers in Psychiatry [Internet]. 2016;7:200. DOI: 10.3389/fpsyt.2016.00200

[115] Tan XW, Lim KWK, Martin D, Tor PC. Effects of electroconvulsive therapy on cognition and quality of life in schizophrenia. Annals, Academy of Medicine, Singapore [Internet]. 2022;**51**(7):400-408. DOI: 10.47102/annals-acadmedsg.202292

[116] Wood H, Cupitt C, Lavender T. The experience of cognitive impairment in people with psychosis. Clinical Psychology & Psychotherapy [Internet]. 2015;**22**(3):193-207. [cited 2024 Dec 10]. DOI: 10.1002/cpp.1878

[117] Riva G, Serino S. Virtual Reality in the Assessment, Understanding and Treatment of Mental Health Disorders [Internet]. 2021. 316 p. Available from: https://books.google.com/books/about/Virtual_Reality_in_the_Assessment_Unders.html?hl=&id=3nzAzgEACAAJ

[118] Fuentes-Claramonte P, Estradé A, Solanes A, Ramella-Cravaro V, Garcia-Leon MA, de Diego-Adeliño J, et al. Biomarkers for psychosis: Are we there yet? Umbrella review of 1478 biomarkers. Schizophrenia Bulletin Open [Internet]. 2024;**5**(1):sgae018. DOI: 10.1093/schizbullopen/sgae018

[119] Smith MJ, Fleming MF, Wright MA, Roberts AG, Humm LB, Olsen D, et al. Virtual reality job interview training and 6-month employment outcomes for individuals with schizophrenia seeking employment. Schizophrenia Research [Internet]. 2015;**166**(1-3):86-91. DOI: 10.1016/j.schres.2015.05.022

[120] Tsang MMY, Man DWK. A virtual reality-based vocational training system (VRVTS) for people with schizophrenia in vocational rehabilitation.

Schizophrenia Research [Internet]. 2013;**144**(1-3):51-62. DOI: 10.1016/j.schres.2012.12.024

[121] Newman-Taylor K, Bentall R. Cognitive behavioural therapy for psychosis: The end of the line or time for a new approach? Psychology and psychotherapy: Theory. Research and Practice [Internet]. 2024;**97**(1):4-18. [cited 2024 Dec 10]. DOI: 10.1111/papt.12498

[122] Kent PL. Evolution of clinical neuropsychology: Four challenges. Applied Neuropsychology Adult [Internet]. 2020;**27**(2):121-133. DOI: 10.1080/23279095.2018.1493483

[123] Glen ET, Hostetter G, Ruff RM, Roebuck-Spencer TM, Denney RL, Perry W, et al. Integrative care models in neuropsychology: A national academy of neuropsychology education paper. Archives of Clinical Neuropsychology [Internet]. 2019;**34**(2):141-151. DOI: 10.1093/arclin/acy092

[124] Péron JA. Challenges and prospects in advancing clinical neuropsychology. Cortex [Internet]. 2024;**179**:261-270. DOI: 10.1016/j.cortex.2024.08.001

Section 3

Clinical Perspectives and Interventions

Chapter 5

The Role of Primary Care in Identifying Early Psychosis

Jared P. Walsh and Barbara C. Walsh

Abstract

Psychological and emotional difficulties are like other medical problems; early signs and symptoms usually occur before serious illnesses develop. As with other medical illnesses, the sooner psychological problems are identified and treated, the less likely they are to disrupt a person's ability to study, work, make friends and be with others. Early identification and treatment can lead to a better prognosis. Primary care can play a major role in recognizing the early warning signs and symptoms and when working collaboratively with Coordinated Specialty Care Clinics for Clinical High Risk of Psychosis or First Episode Psychosis can help facilitate this improved prognosis.

Keywords: psychosis, clinical high risk, warning signs, early identification, primary care

1. Introduction

Psychosis is a mental disorder that usually appears in late adolescence or early adulthood and can have a broad impact on an individual's ability to live a productive life. It is often characterized by delusions, hallucinations, and other cognitive difficulties, resulting in a lifelong struggle. Psychosis can have a major effect on the total burden of disease to the public. One psychotic disorder called Schizophrenia is one of the most disabling and costly of diseases. It is the most severe mental disorder, often creating continuous disability for a lifetime. Its prevalence is about 1% or between 0.27 and 0.83% of the population and it is the fifth leading cause of disability and premature mortality among all medical disorders [1] and has been estimated that the total lifetime cost for a single case of schizophrenia is greater than $10,000,000 [2]. Twenty-five percent of all hospital admissions and disability payments in the U.S. are accounted for by patients with severe mental illness, most of them for schizophrenia or other psychotic disorders and meta-analyses have found that schizophrenia exacts a 25 year reduction in life expectancy [3].

The high cost, both to the patient and to society, has led to an effort to understand the potential for early detection and intervention. It takes approximately 1.5 years between onset of symptoms and diagnosis of psychosis in young adults [4]. Even more concerning is that young individuals with psychosis are approximately twelve times as likely to commit suicide as the general population [5]. There has been significant work trying to understand the risk factors for the development of schizophrenia. One of the strongest risk factors remains family history, with a strong genetic linkage. Having a first-degree relative with schizophrenia or a related disorder significantly increases an individual's risk [6]. In addition, substance misuse, particularly cannabis misuse, has been strongly correlated with psychosis risk if started at a younger age [7]. The duration of untreated psychosis, defined as the time from the first psychotic symptom to the initiation of appropriate treatment, has been associated as a predictor of long-term outcomes in schizophrenia, with the longer the duration, the poorer the outcome. The mechanism is hypothesized to be a toxic effect through some as yet unconfirmed psychological or neurological mechanism [8].

One major consequence of this delay is the potential exacerbation of symptoms. If treatment is delayed, emerging delusions or hallucinations may become more entrenched, and negative symptoms—such as social withdrawal, anhedonia, or apathy—can worsen. This symptom intensification increases the likelihood of crisis episodes that may require hospitalization. Additionally, prolonged untreated psychosis can contribute to higher levels of distress and suffering for the patient, potentially fueling secondary problems such as depression and suicidal ideation. This is then complicated by functional and social decline- such as disruption in the individual's ability to maintain employment, fulfill school obligations, or nurture relationships. As an example, a young adult attending college, might withdraw from classes or lose academic scholarships if emerging delusions and paranoia go unnoticed for several months. Similar patterns can occur in the workforce, as difficulty concentrating and shifts in behavior may jeopardize job performance. When psychotic symptoms remain untreated, patients are at heightened risk for losing important social networks and support systems, making functional recovery more difficult once treatment eventually begins [9]. In addition, psychotic disorders are associated with elevated rates of comorbid medical conditions, such as cardiovascular disease and metabolic syndrome with delayed intervention depriving individuals of valuable support in controlling these risk factors [10].

A systematic review confirmed that there is in fact, a modest association between the duration of untreated psychosis and outcomes, which supports efforts for early intervention programs [11]. This leads to better symptom control, improved functional outcomes, and enhanced quality of life. Other trials have established that an early intervention program is in fact feasible and can successfully reduce the duration of untreated psychosis [12]. As early identification can improve outcomes in patients with this high-burden disease, primary care represents an underutilized opportunity for intervention.

In the US Healthcare System, 50.3% of all physician visits are with a primary care physician [13]. While primary care physicians (PCPs) make up only approximately 1/3 of the US physician workforce, they deliver the majority of ambulatory visits [14]. Within those visits, it is estimated that PCPs deliver mental health care for approximately 60% of patients with a behavioral health condition [15]. This combination makes PCPs a key target for screening programs for behavioral health and substance misuse. This role has been endorsed by the United States Preventative Services Taskforce (USPSTF), which recommends screening for depression and substance misuse in the primary care setting. Given this and the long-term relationship PCPs establish with patients, and often their families, they are well positioned to identify changes in medical and behavioral health – and importantly, the ability to distinguish when a somatic symptom is actually a sign of a behavioral health condition rather than a routine medical condition.

2. Understanding early psychosis

Early psychosis refers to the initial manifestations or prodromal stages of serious mental illness, such as schizophrenia-spectrum disorders or other psychotic conditions. While full-blown psychosis is easier to recognize—typically involving fixed delusions or overt hallucinations—the earliest symptoms can be mild or ambiguous, presenting as changes in affect, behavior, or cognition. PCPs are likely to see a variety of presentations, including subtle or attenuated positive symptoms, negative and affective symptoms, disorganized thinking or behavior, and regression or stalls in childhood development. The early onset of hallucinations can be subtle, such as a patient reporting faint whispers, their name called when no one is around, or seeing fleeting shadows. Early development of paranoia can present as vague suspicions of people talking about them behind their backs or minor conspiracies – all behaviors that can be confused with adolescent development. Patients themselves may question the validity of these beliefs or experiences, making it seem as though it may just be a more benign condition if a high index of suspicion is not maintained. Alternatively, patients may withdraw from activities they once enjoyed or start spending more time alone. A student with previously good grades may begin failing exams or missing assignments; an adult may struggle to keep pace with routine work tasks. These changes can easily be misattributed to other behavioral health conditions such as depression or anxiety, which frequently co-present with early psychosis.

Multiple studies have shown that there is an increase in contact between patients with early psychosis and their PCPs in years prior to diagnosis of schizophrenia and that the increase in contact can lead to a reduction in the duration of untreated psychosis [16, 17]. However, another study has shown that failure to recognize the symptoms of early psychosis by PCPs leads to an increased duration of untreated psychosis, making PCP education a key priority [18]. Thus, it is reasonable to hypothesize that PCPs well-versed in the identification of early psychosis can intervene to reduce the duration of untreated psychosis, leading to improved outcomes in a disease with a high personal and socioeconomic cost.

A UK study looked into identifying the pattern of symptoms seen in primary care offices for patients with early psychosis [19]. They identified the following (chart) (**Table 1**) [19]:

Specific early warning signs of psychosis in young people that can be identified by PCPs are:

- Increased difficulty at school or work
- Withdrawal from friends or family
- Difficulty concentrating or thinking clearly
- Suspiciousness or mistrust of others
- Changes in the way things look or sound
- Odd thinking or behavior
- Emotional outbursts or lack of emotion
- Poor personal hygiene.

Symptom group	FEP patients (n = 3045)		Matched participants (n = 12,180)		Crude odds ratio (95% CI)‡	Adjusted odds ratio‡* (95% CI)
	$n^{\dagger}$	5-year prevalence (%)	$n^{\dagger}$	5-year prevalence (%)		
Psychological symptom						
Mood-related symptom	1473	48.4	1275	10.5	10.1 (9.12, 11.3)	7.60 (6.75, 8.56)
'Neurotic' symptom	1133	37.2	1106	9.1	6.54 (5.89, 7.27)	4.87 (4.35, 5.47)
Behavioral change	490	16.1	657	5.4	3.53 (3.08, 4.05)	2.67 (2.30, 3.09)
Change in volition	394	12.9	923	7.6	1.88 (1.64, 2.16)	1.33 (1.14, 1.55)
Perceptual problem	162	5.3	5	0.04	130 (53.7, 313)	112 (44.4, 283)
Cognitive change	38	1.3	30	0.3	5.41 (3.35, 8.75)	3.80 (2.04, 7.09)
Substance misuse	338	11.1	134	1.1	13.0 (10.4, 16.4)	8.09 (6.36, 10.3)
Physical symptom	939	30.8	1926	15.8	2.70 (2.43, 2.99)	1.80 (1.61, 2.02)

FEP first episode psychosis, CI confidence interval.
†Number of individuals with recorded symptom in the 5-year period before the index date.
*‡Conditional logistic regression analyses with cluster-robust variance estimator. *Adjusted for smoking, alcohol consumption, BMI morbidity burden, and specific co-morbid conditions (including respiratory condition, musculoskeletal pain, and injury and major trauma), in addition to matched year of birth (age), gender, and practice.*

Table 1.
Pattern of symptoms before a diagnosis of first episode psychosis: A latent class analysis of UK primary care electronic health records. BMC Medicine. 2019;17:227.

A PCP who identifies these symptoms should use a validated scale to screen for early psychosis.

3. Screening for early psychosis

There are short, quick screeners available to assess for attenuated psychosis symptoms. One of these screeners, the PRIME Screen, is twelve questions that can be used as a self-report or can be administered by a lay person. Scoring standards are provided which alert the professional whether a specialized evaluation is warranted. The questionnaire has been validated in multinational samples. It is available in open domain by authors Drs. Thomas McGlashan, Tandy Miller and Scott Woods of the PRIME Clinic - Yale School of Medicine. If an individual meets the criteria based on a score of six on any one item or three fives on any items, then they should be referred for a specialized assessment. These assessments are conducted by a professional specifically certified in their administration and interpretation. These professionals are usually located in Coordinated Specialty Care Clinics for either Clinical High Risk or First Episode Psychosis. A listing by state of these clinics, or professional credentialed in the specialized assessments, can be found by referring to the substance Abuse. (SAMHSA) early serious mental illness website or by consulting thesipstraining.com website (**Table 2**).

To introduce the screen to respondents, explain that questionnaires usually ask about different kinds of experiences like mood and anxiety, this one asks about

PRIME Screen

Date: □□ / □□ / □□ AGE: □□ Gender: M F

Please read the attached information sheet before completing this questionnaire.

The following screen asks about your personal experiences. It asks about your sensory, psychological, emotional, and social experiences. Some of these questions may seem to relate directly to your experiences and others may not.

Based on your experiences within the past year, please indicate how much you agree or disagree with the following statements.

Please read each question carefully and circle the answer that best describes your experience. Please answer all questions.

	Within the past year:						
	0 definitely disagree	**1 somewhat disagree**	**2 slightly disagree**	**3 not sure**	**4 slightly agree**	**5 somewhat agree**	**6 definitely agree**
Within the past year:	Definitely disagree	Somewhat disagree	Slightly disagree	Not sure	Slightly agree	Somewhat agree	Definitely agree
1. I think that I have felt that there are odd or unusual things going on that I can't explain.	0	1	2	3	4	5	6
2. I think that I might be able to predict the future.	0	1	2	3	4	5	6
3. I may have felt that there could possibly be something interrupting or controlling my thoughts, feelings, or actions.	0	1	2	3	4	5	6
4. I have had the experience of doing something differently because of my superstitions.	0	1	2	3	4	5	6
5. I think that I may get confused at times whether something I experience or perceive may be real or may be just part of my imagination or dreams	0	1	2	3	4	5	6
6. I have thought that it might be possible that other people can read my mind, or that I can read other's minds	0	1	2	3	4	5	6
7. I wonder if people may be planning to hurt me or even may be about to hurt me.	0	1	2	3	4	5	6

8. I believe that I have special natural or supernatural gifts beyond my talents and natural strengths.	0	1	2	3	4	5	6
9. I think I might feel like my mind is "playing tricks" on me.	0	1	2	3	4	5	6
10. I have had the experience of hearing faint or fear sounds of people or a person mumbling or talking when there is no one near me.	0	1	2	3	4	5	6
11. I think that I may hear my own thoughts being said out loud.	0	1	2	3	4	5	6
12. I have been concerned that I might be "going crazy".	0	1	2	3	4	5	6
Version A July 2004						HIC 26895	

Table 2.
Pattern of symptoms before a diagnosis of first episode psychosis: A latent class analysis of UK primary care electronic health records. BMC Medicine. 2019;17:227.

things that can cause worry or stress. Explain that if you experience some of these things, further evaluation of those experiences might be helpful for you and your treatment. Ask the respondent to complete the questionnaire in a private, confidential space. Read the directions to the respondent. Offer to read the questions aloud if the respondent has difficulties reading or responding independently. Provide simple explanations or synonyms as needed and avoid elaboration or in-depth discussion of items.

This questionnaire can be implanted in primary care in a similar manner to other behavioral health conditions, such as the PHQ-2/PHQ-9, AUDIT, and GAD screening tools. These tools are often available in the electronic medical records (EMR), and this tool could also be incorporated. While the time pressures on PCPs continue to escalate, utilization of team-based care models can help alleviate the strain of additional screening. However, PCPs need to be prepared for the next steps in discussing positive screens with patients and families. This will involve a focus on communication skills, as well as describing next steps.

4. Managing a positive screen

The steps involved in managing a positive screen include a focus on patient-centered communication, patient and family education, and sharing of resources to build a comprehensive evaluation plan. Communicating the results of the screen with a patient and their family or support persons can be complicated given the potentially life-altering nature of the diagnosis and stigma associated with psychosis. A patient-centered approach with a focus on empathy, respect, and flexibility in communication is key to maintain the physician-patient relationship and trust in the healthcare system while minimizing the potential trauma to the patient receiving the diagnosis.

Physicians should approach this conversation in a similar manner as they would when delivering bad or life altering news. There are several recognized protocols for approaching these conversations, such as SPIKES, ABCDE or BREAKS models [20]. As the SPIKES protocol can be used with children and adults, we will review that here [20]. The SPIKES protocol consists of six steps: Setting, Perception, Invitation, Knowledge, Emotions, and Strategy and Summary [20].

The *Setting* refers to setting up the area where the conversation will take place, such as arranging for a private area, sitting near the patient with clear eye contact, ensuring support items like tissues and water are available, and limiting distractions like pagers, phones, electronic medical records. In addition, you should offer to have the patient invite any support persons to the conversation while also ensuring the patient is allowed to feel less vulnerable (e.g. allow the patient to change from an examination gown to their own clothing).

Perception refers to understanding the patient's knowledge of what has happened so far. Physicians should utilize open-ended questions to evaluate the patient's understanding of illness – in this case what screening is, how it is different from making a diagnosis, and what psychosis is. This provides an opportunity to correct misunderstandings, misinformation, or unrealistic expectations.

Invitation allows you to provide the patient with some measure of control during this conversation by asking permission to share information. This also provides an opportunity to explore how much information the patient wants.

The *Knowledge* step is where the physician briefly summarizes the events leading up to this point. This would include the symptoms that triggered the screening and what information was gathered during the screening. This step also provides an opportunity for a warning statement to help lessen the shock. Physician should ensure to use non-medical terminology and avoid any medical/technical jargon during the conversation. Teach back to confirm understanding as well as offering the opportunity to ask questions are also key aspects of this step.

Emotional reactions are a normal part of this conversation and can also be a source of stress for both physician and patient. The *Emotions* step provides some guidance on managing these reactions. It is important to pause during the conversation and address the emotion. A successful strategy is simply naming the emotion and inquiring further about the patient's response. Utilize empathy statements here and validate your patient's responses to demonstrate to the patient that you understand their emotions are important and valid.

Strategy and Summary is the final step. In this step you summarize the news, invite the patient to return with questions as they arise in the future, and set a plan for follow-up. The plan for follow-up will help the patient understand what additional tests or referral to other providers are needed which we will now pivot to discuss.

Generally interventions for the evaluation and treatment of early psychosis are not likely to be available in a patient's usual community treatment setting. As the primary care physician, you will need to refer your patient to a center with expertise in coordinated specialty care for first episode psychosis (FEP) or clinical high risk for psychosis (CHR). The treatment goals in these centers are to make a diagnosis, reduce symptoms and disability, improve social and occupational/educational functioning, improve quality of life, and to prevent or delay further progression of psychosis. One such center is the PRIME Clinic in New Haven, CT which is the first CHR clinic organized in North America. This center specializes in the assessment of CHR in persons aged 12–25 and treats patients throughout North America, while also providing training and certification of clinicians working to provide these services in other geographic areas.

When patients are referred to a CHR/FEP center, they can expect several steps. There is typically an initial phone screen/online screening form that either the patient, family member, or clinician could complete. The center will then schedule the patient for their initial assessment utilizing the Structured Interview of Psychosis-risk Syndromes (SIPS). The SIPS is a series of questions administered by a certified behavioral health clinician that reviews a patients history and the patient's experiences/symptoms. This interview can last from 45 minutes to 2 hours and can be completed in person or via telehealth. If a patient is under the age of 18, a parent or legal guardian will need to be present for part of the assessment. After the completion of this assessment, the results are communicated to the patient and treatment options can be discussed.

Patients may have more specific questions about early psychosis and what specific treatments are available. The primary care physician is not expected to be an expert in this area but can utilize the below information to help begin educating the patient.

The benefits of early intervention are to foster a strong therapeutic relationship, to increase the likelihood that the individuals will accept treatment, and to allow for rapid access to treatment to reduce the DUP to improve long term prognosis. Patients may also ask questions about what they should expect, such as "when might we expect the symptoms to get worse?" Generally, research has shown that the highest risk of conversion to psychosis is in the first 1–2 years but can take as long as 10-years [21]. Patients will need close monitoring for progression to psychosis during this time and may be started on second-generation antipsychotic medications. Co-existing conditions such as depression and anxiety can be managed by the behavioral health team as well. Talk therapy, including individual therapies such as cognitive behavioral therapy as well as family intervention therapy, are a key component of the care plan as well. Rehabilitation programs to help patients build confidence and skills to cope with their illness and remain independent are also offered to many patients.

5. Case examples

A 14-year-old female completed the PRIME Screen and endorsed that she had the experience of a tactile illusion when she sat at the kitchen table in her home. A cold wave would come over her. When queried what she made of this experience she stated that she thought it was the ghost of her dead grandmother coming to comfort her. While she was not distressed by this experience, in fact she reported feeling comforted by it, she was spending more and more time sitting at the kitchen table waiting for Grandma to come and was not going to school or being social with her friends. It was interfering with her daily functioning. She was referred to the PRIME Clinic for the Structured Interview for Psychosis-risk syndromes (SIPS) and did meet criteria for being at risk of developing a psychotic disorder. She entered specialty care receiving psychoeducation for her and her parents regarding early warning signs of risk, Cognitive Behavior therapy for early psychosis, medication management of her coexisting anxiety and follow-up evaluations to monitor for progression or improvement of her symptoms. The patient's symptoms remitted after the first year of treatment, medication was discontinued, and she was followed for an additional year with supportive therapy.

A 16-year-old young male was given the PRIME Screen when he reported to his PCP that he was hearing things and was socially isolating from his friends. He was referred to the PRIME Clinic for the SIPS and did meet criteria for being at risk for developing a psychotic disorder. He entered specialty care and received the psychoeducation, The CBT-ep, participated in a support group for young people with similar experiences and was monitored for progression or improvement of his symptoms. He responded to the treatment very quickly and remitted within 9 months and was then offered the supportive therapy until the end of the two-year treatment protocol. Treatment is typically offered for a two-year period as the first 2 years after the onset of at risk symptoms is when the risk for conversion to psychosis is at the highest.

6. Conclusion

Primary care physicians play a pivotal role in recognizing the early, often subtle signs of psychosis. By establishing systematic screening protocols, employing validated tools, and building strong referral networks with mental health specialists, PCPs can meaningfully reduce the duration of untreated psychosis and improve patient trajectories. Collaborative care models—integrating mental and physical health services—underscore the value of a team-based, person-centered approach that aligns with the values of modern primary care.

In the face of growing evidence that early intervention can alter the course of psychotic disorders, PCPs have an unprecedented opportunity to intervene at a critical juncture. By engaging in continuous education, leveraging technology, and embracing integrated behavioral health approaches, primary care practices can create a more responsive, holistic environment where patients with early psychosis receive timely, evidence-based, and compassionate care. By working together with the coordinated specialty care services available, professionals create a strong network for early identification and intervention of serious mental illness in adolescents and young adults.

Author details

Jared P. Walsh[1] and Barbara C. Walsh[2*]

1 Medicine, Internal Medicine, Rutgers New Jersey Medical School, Newark, New Jersey, United States

2 PRIME Clinic at Yale School of Medicine, New Haven, CT, United States

*Address all correspondence to: barbara.walsh@yale.edu

References

[1] Eaton WW. Evidence for university and uniformity of schizophrenia around the world: Assessment and implications. In: Gattaz WF, Hafner H, editors. Search for the Causes of Schizophrenia. Vol. IV. Steinkopf: Springer; 1999. pp. 21-33

[2] Rupp A, Keith SJ. The costs of schizophrenia. Psychiatric Clinics of North America. 1993;**16**(2):413-423

[3] Parks J, Svendsen D, Singer P, Foti ME, Mauer B. Morbidity and mortality in people with serious mental illness. Alexandria, VA: National association of state mental health program directors (NASMHPD) Medical Directors Council; 2006;**25**(4):1-87

[4] Perkins DO, Gu H, Boteva K, Lieberman JA. Relationship between duration of untreated psychosis and outcome in first-episode schizophrenia: A critical review and meta-analysis. American Journal of Psychiatry. 2005;**162**(10):1785-1804

[5] Dutta R, Murray RM, Hotopf M, Allardyce J, Jones PB, Boydell J. Reassessing the long-term risk of suicide after a first episode of psychosis. Archives of General Psychiatry. 2010;**67**(12):1230-1237

[6] Freedman R. Schizophrenia. New England Journal of Medicine. 2003;**349**(18):1738-1749

[7] Di Forti M et al. Proportion of patients in South London with first-episode psychosis attributable to use of high-potency cannabis: A case-control study. The Lancet Psychiatry. 2015;**2**(3):233-238

[8] Sheitman B, Lieberman JA. The natural history and pathophysiology of treatment resistant schizophrenia. Journal of Psychiatric Research. 1998;**32**(3-4):143-150

[9] Horan WP, Subotnik KL, Snyder KS, Nuechterlein KH. Do recent-onset schizophrenia patients experience a "social network crisis"? Psychiatry. 2010;**73**(3):172-183

[10] De Hert M, Schreurs V, Vancampfort D, Van Winkel R. Metabolic syndrome in people with schizophrenia: A review. World Psychiatry. 2009;**8**(1):15-22. DOI: 10.1002/j.2051-5545.2009.tb00199.x. Erratum in: World Psychiatry. 2011;10(1):78

[11] Marshall M, Lewis S, Lockwood A, Drake R, Jones P, Croudace T. Association between duration of untreated psychosis and outcome in cohorts of first-episode patients: A systematic review. Archives of General Psychiatry. 2005;**62**(9):975-983

[12] Larsen TK, McGlashan TH, Johannessen JO, Friis S, Guldberg C, Haah U, et al. Shortened duration of untreated first episode of psychosis: Changes in patient characteristics at treatment. The American Journal of Psychiatry. 2001:1581917-1581919

[13] Santo L, Kang K. National hospital ambulatory medical care survey: 2019 National summary tables. 2023

[14] Association of American Medical Colleges (AAMC). 2022 Physician Specialty Data Report. 2022

[15] Butler DJ, Fons D, Fisher T, et al. A review of the benefits and limitations of a primary care-embedded psychiatric consultation service in a medically underserved setting. International Journal of Psychiatry in Medicine. 2018;**53**:415-426

[16] Nørgaard H, Søndergaard Pedersen H, Fenger-Grøn M, Mors O, Nordentoft M, Vestergaard M, et al. Increased use of primary care during 6 years of prodromal schizophrenia. Acta Psychiatrica Scandinavica. 2016;**134**:225-233

[17] Skeate A, Jackson C, Birchwood M, Jones C. Duration of untreated psychosis and pathways to care in first-episode psychosis. Investigation of help-seeking behaviour in primary care. The British Journal of Psychiatry. 2002;**43**:s73-s77

[18] Platz C, Umbricht DS, Cattapan-Ludewig K, Dvorsky D, Arbach D, Brenner HD, et al. Help-seeking pathways in early psychosis. Social Psychiatry and Psychiatric Epidemiology. 2006;**41**:967-974

[19] Chen Y, Farooq S, Edwards J, et al. Patterns of symptoms before a diagnosis of first episode psychosis: A latent class analysis of UK primary care electronic health records. BMC Medicine. 2019;**17**:227

[20] Berkey FJ, Wiedemer JP, Vithalani ND. Delivering bad or life-altering news. American Family Physician. 2018;**98**(2):99-104

[21] Nelson B, Yuen HP, Wood SJ, et al. JAMA Psychiatry. 2013;**70**(8):793-802. DOI: 10.1001/jamapsychiatry.2013.1270

Chapter 6

Psychoactive Substance-Induced Psychotic Disorder

Elif Küçük and Feride Uysal

Abstract

Substance-induced psychotic disorder (SIPD) is characterized by delusions and hallucinations occurring during or shortly after the intoxication or withdrawal phases of psychoactive substance (PAS) use. It represents a significant challenge within psychiatry, accounting for a notable proportion of first-episode psychosis cases. The prevalence of SIPD is influenced by the type, dose, and duration of substance use, as well as genetic and environmental factors. Diagnostic criteria from DSM-5 and ICD-10 emphasize the temporal link between substance use and psychotic symptoms, the exclusion of primary psychotic disorders, and the associated distress or functional impairment. The neurobiological mechanisms of SIPD differ across substances, implicating dopaminergic, glutamatergic, and serotonergic systems in its pathogenesis. Cannabinoids affect the endocannabinoid system, while methamphetamine and cocaine disrupt monoamine transporter function. Risk factors include genetic predisposition, polysubstance use, and comorbid psychiatric disorders. Clinical presentations vary, with cannabinoids often causing paranoid delusions, synthetic cannabinoids inducing severe psychotic symptoms, and methamphetamine and cocaine leading to tactile hallucinations and aggression. Treatment requires an integrated approach combining pharmacological and psychosocial strategies. Second-generation antipsychotics, such as clozapine and olanzapine, are preferred for their ability to reduce psychotic symptoms and substance craving. Cognitive-behavioral therapy and motivational interviewing effectively address both psychosis and substance use. Group therapies further enhance adherence and recovery by improving social functioning. Accurate diagnosis and individualized treatment are essential to prevent SIPD from progressing into chronic psychotic disorders like schizophrenia. Future research should focus on the complex interactions between genetic and environmental factors and the development of targeted, evidence-based treatments for SIPD.

Keywords: substance-induced psychotic disorder, psychoactive substances, psychotic symptoms, substance use, schizophrenia

1. Introduction

Schizophrenia spectrum and other psychotic disorders are defined by impairments in five core domains: delusions, hallucinations, disorganized thinking, disorganized behavior, and negative symptoms [1]. These features are crucial for accurate diagnosis and for monitoring the clinical course of the disorder. Substance use disorders are frequently observed in cases of psychotic disorders, adding complexity to their management. While the prevalence of substance use disorders in the general population is approximately 15%, this rate can rise to as high as 50% among individuals with psychotic disorders [2].

Psychoactive substances (PAS) are chemical compounds that exert significant stimulatory or suppressive effects on the central nervous system, leading to various disturbances in mental state, mood, perception, behavior, and motor functions [3]. Research clearly shows that the use of PAS can contribute to the emergence of various psychiatric disorders, especially substance-induced psychotic disorders (SIPD) [4]. Substance use disorders and psychotic disorders are significant public health concerns, often co-occurring and sharing common neurobiological foundations. Understanding the factors influencing this comorbidity is critical for accurate diagnosis and the development of effective treatment approaches [5]. Notably, the fact that substance-induced psychotic disorders can turn into long-term psychotic disorders like schizophrenia or bipolar disorder shows how important it is to get diagnosed and treated quickly [5].

The diagnosis of SIPD was first introduced in 1994 within the classification system of the *Diagnostic and Statistical Manual of Mental Disorders* (DSM)-IV [6]. This diagnostic category was developed to distinguish substance-related psychotic disorders from primary psychotic disorders and was shaped based on recommendations from the Substance Use Disorders Work Group. The diagnostic criteria for SIPD were mostly kept the same in DSM-5, but it was made clear that delusions and/or hallucinations must be clinically significant and need help [7]. According to the DSM-5, SIPD is defined as a mental disorder characterized by delusions and/or hallucinations occurring during or shortly after the intoxication or withdrawal phase of a PAS. The symptoms must not be better explained by delirium or another psychotic disorder [8]. To be diagnosed with SIPD, a person must not have had any psychotic symptoms before using PAS, start showing them after using PAS, and be able to show a clear link between the psychosis and the substance. Furthermore, the psychotic symptoms must be explainable by the effects of the specific substance used [9].

2. Substance-induced psychotic disorder: Definition, diagnostic criteria, and differential diagnosis

SIPD is defined by distinct diagnostic criteria. The presence of delusions and/or hallucinations is considered the primary hallmark of this disorder. History, physical examination, or laboratory findings must indicate that these symptoms developed during or immediately after substance intoxication, withdrawal, or medication use and that the implicated substance/medication can trigger such symptoms. This disorder should not be better explained by another psychotic disorder. For example, symptoms that were there before using drugs or alcohol and last for a long time (like a month or more) after acute withdrawal or severe intoxication are over, or a history of recurring psychotic episodes that are not related to the drugs or alcohol, could be signs of a different psychotic disorder. Additionally, the symptoms should not occur exclusively during delirium and must cause clinically significant distress or substantial impairment in social, occupational, or other critical areas of functioning. These criteria are crucial for accurately identifying SIPD and distinguishing it from other psychotic disorders [1].

In the 10th edition of the *International Classification of Diseases* (ICD-10), SIPD is categorized under "Mental and Behavioral Disorders Due to Psychoactive Substance

Use," emphasizing that symptoms should partially resolve within 1 month and fully resolve within 6 months [10]. The challenges in definitively diagnosing SIPD based on classification system criteria raise concerns about the reliability of its epidemiological data. Additionally, regional variations in substance use patterns and prevalence contribute to discrepancies in SIPD incidence across studies. For instance, data from the Danish Psychiatric Central Research Register reported the incidence of cannabis-induced psychotic disorder as 2.7 cases per 100,000 individuals per year [11]. In a 2013 study by Weibell and colleagues, this rate was found to be 6.5 [12]. According to DSM-5, SIPD is estimated to account for 7–25% of cases presenting with a first psychotic episode [13]. Furthermore, it has been suggested that approximately half of individuals using psychoactive substances may exhibit psychotic symptoms at some point [14].

Psychotic disorders can be associated with intoxication from alcohol, cannabis, hallucinogens (including phencyclidine and related substances), inhalants, sedatives, hypnotics, anxiolytics, stimulants (including cocaine), and other or unknown substances. Similarly, psychotic disorders may also emerge during withdrawal from alcohol, sedatives, hypnotics, anxiolytics, and other or unknown substances [15–17]. In the literature, cannabis and methamphetamine have been reported to have the strongest associations with the development of psychosis [16, 18]. The prevalence of cannabis use among new treatment admissions increased from 29% in 2003 to 46% in 2014 [19]. Scandinavia, particularly Denmark, Norway, and Sweden, has witnessed a similar trend, with cannabis use significantly increasing since 2010 [20]. Additionally, clinical follow-up reports are showing an increasing number of patients with synthetic cannabinoid (SC)-induced psychotic disorder [21].

The distinction between SIPD and primary psychosis is critical for understanding the course of the illness and planning appropriate treatment. Accurate differential diagnosis of psychotic disorders in the early stages is crucial for determining prognosis [22]. Misdiagnosing SIPD can lead to unnecessary use of antipsychotics and adverse social and occupational outcomes [23]. Therefore, there is a need for early and accurate differential diagnosis, as well as the use of evidence-based and clear criteria to prevent diagnostic uncertainties in psychotic disorders [24]. The similar clinical features of primary psychotic disorders and SIPD, combined with the high prevalence of substance use in both groups, make differential diagnosis challenging [25]. In a study involving patients with first-episode psychosis, substance use disorder was identified as the most common cause of diagnostic uncertainty [26]. Although the relationship between substance use and psychotic disorders has been established, its nature is complex, and a clear cause-and-effect connection has not yet been fully elucidated. Establishing a definitive diagnosis of SIPD at the onset is challenging and often requires longitudinal follow-up to clarify the diagnosis [27].

3. Etiology and risk factors in substance-induced psychotic disorders

Studies aiming to elucidate the onset of SIPD have significantly contributed to the neurobiological theories of schizophrenia and other psychotic disorders. It has been shown that the mechanisms through which each PAS induces psychotic disorders vary and may explain different models of schizophrenia pathogenesis [15]. For example, Lysergic Acid Diethylamide (LSD) supports the serotonergic model, amphetamines and cocaine align with the dopamine hypothesis, and phencyclidine and ketamine provide evidence for the glutamatergic model [28–30]. Nonetheless, the psychotogenic effects of PAS are most commonly associated with dopaminergic activity. Mesolimbic and mesocortical dopaminergic circuits play roles in both reward mechanisms and the development of psychotic symptoms. Substances that increase dopamine levels in these circuits are believed to lead to symptoms resembling schizophrenia [31].

The discovery of the psychomimetic effects of cannabinoids has spurred research into the endocannabinoid system, but the neurobiological processes underlying the relationship between cannabis and psychosis remain incompletely understood [32]. The primary psychoactive component of cannabis, Δ9-tetrahydrocannabinol (THC), acts as a partial agonist at cannabinoid type 1 (CB1R) and type 2 (CB2R) receptors [33]. CB1R is predominantly concentrated in central nervous system regions associated with mood and memory, while CB2R is primarily located in peripheral immune cells [34]. The psychomimetic effects of THC occur *via* CB1R activation, which influences the glutamatergic and dopaminergic systems implicated in the etiology of schizophrenia. Acute exposure to Δ9-THC increases dopaminergic activity, whereas chronic use is associated with reduced dopamine synthesis capacity [35]. These changes are thought to mirror mechanisms observed in schizophrenia. Furthermore, the association of chronic cannabis use with persistent impairments in memory and cognitive function is explained by a reduction in CB1R density in the responsible brain regions [36]. SCs, on the other hand, act as full agonists at CB1R, leading to significantly stronger psychoactive effects compared to THC [37]. Researchers have reported that components like JHW-018 in synthetic cannabinoids can induce psychosis [38].

Methamphetamine and cocaine block the transporters of dopamine, norepinephrine, and serotonin. This raises monoamine levels, which is thought to play a part in the development of psychotic disorders [39]. In contrast, 3,4-methylenedioxymethamphetamine (MDMA or ecstasy) disrupts serotonergic and dopaminergic systems [40].

Risk factors for SIPD include the type of substance, route of administration, dosage, duration of use, age, sex, genetic predisposition, family history of psychotic disorders, comorbid psychiatric disorders, and polysubstance use [41]. Chronic and heavy substance use has been identified as a significant risk factor, with polysubstance use being the strongest predictor of psychosis [42, 43]. Cannabinoids are reported to more strongly trigger psychotic symptoms in individuals predisposed to psychosis, with genetic susceptibility and environmental risk factors further increasing this likelihood [44, 45]. In recent studies, it has been emphasized that the relationship between cannabinoid use and psychosis is based on multifactorial risk factors and that two different gene-environment interactions play a role [46]. The association between other PAS and psychosis is similarly multifactorial, with methamphetamine frequency of use and addiction severity identified as primary risk factors. Genetic predisposition, family history of psychotic disorders, and a history of trauma have also been noted to increase the risk [47]. Cocaine-induced psychosis risk has been linked to psychosis vulnerability, sex, duration of use, route of administration, and dose. Continued use has been reported to result in more rapid and severe development of psychosis [48].

4. Clinical features of substance-induced psychotic disorders

The most common psychotic symptoms in SIPD are delusions and hallucinations that develop following substance use. Symptoms such as agitation and aggression are also frequently observed [49]. The literature reports variable findings regarding the clinical differences between SIPD and primary psychotic disorders. The most consistent finding is that SIPD patients tend to experience fewer negative symptoms compared to those with primary psychotic disorders [50]. In terms of positive symptoms, SIPD is often characterized by paranoid delusions and psychotic features that vary depending on the specific PAS used. For instance, cannabis is associated with paranoid delusions, LSD with visual hallucinations, and N-methyl-D-aspartate (NMDA) receptor antagonists with negative and cognitive symptoms [18, 23].

The use of Δ9-THC has been shown to induce positive symptoms such as paranoid delusions, hallucinations, and disorganized speech; negative symptoms including affective flattening, social withdrawal, and psychomotor retardation; perceptual changes; cognitive impairments; as well as increased anxiety and euphoria [51]. SCs have been reported to cause psychotic symptoms such as auditory and visual hallucinations, paranoid delusions, thought blocking, and disorganized speech [52]. In addition, SCs are associated with the various effects, including cognitive impairments, memory issues, anxiety, agitation, and suicidal ideation [53]. Compared to cannabinoids, SCs cause more severe mental deterioration and psychotic disorders [38]. In patients with SC-induced psychotic disorder, positive symptoms have been found to be similar to those observed in schizophrenia, while negative symptoms appear less prominent, and certain cognitive impairments are more pronounced [54].

The use of MDMA has been reported to cause symptoms such as paranoid delusions, anxiety, depressive symptoms, memory and attention deficits, aggression, and violent behavior [55]. Symptoms of psychotic disorders linked to ecstasy use are similar to those of primary psychotic disorders, but visual hallucinations and skewed perceptions are more common in psychotic disorders caused by ecstasy [56]. In patients with methamphetamine-induced acute psychotic disorder, positive symptoms such as delusions and hallucinations are predominant, while negative symptoms, Schneider's first-rank symptoms, and cognitive impairments are rarely observed [57]. A systematic review reported the most common symptoms in methamphetamine-induced acute psychotic disorder as persecutory delusions (84%), auditory hallucinations (69%), visual hallucinations (65%), and violent or aggressive behavior (53%). Less commonly reported symptoms included disorganized behavior, depression, referential delusions, tactile hallucinations, and inappropriate affect [58]. Studies examining the phenomenology of methamphetamine-induced acute psychotic disorder highlight that visual and tactile hallucinations (e.g., the sensation of insects crawling under the skin) are more prevalent compared to other psychotic disorders, and methamphetamine-induced acute psychotic disorder has a high tendency to become chronic [59]. In chronic methamphetamine-induced psychosis, negative symptoms, Schneider's first-rank symptoms, and cognitive impairments often resemble those seen in schizophrenia [47].

In cocaine-induced psychotic disorders, the most common symptom is paranoid delusions, followed by auditory hallucinations. Less frequently, specific symptoms such as visual and tactile hallucinations, formication, and delusions centered on substance use behavior are observed [60]. While hallucinations are frequent in cocaine-induced psychosis, thought disorders, bizarre delusions, and negative symptoms are rare, severe hallucinations have been reported to resolve rapidly [61].

5. Treatment of substance-induced psychotic disorder

Substance use is steadily increasing worldwide, resulting in the widespread prevalence of substance-related disorders that pose significant psychological and social challenges. Given the potential for these disorders to progress into severe psychotic illnesses at later stages, it is crucial to ensure accurate and effective diagnosis and treatment.

In the treatment of SIPD:

- Reducing and ultimately eliminating the craving for substance use,
- Restoring the individual's functionality,
- Preventing complications and the risk of relapse.

To reach these goals, a coordinated plan is put in place that includes both drug-based treatments and supportive ones, such as counseling, rehabilitation, and programs that help people who are struggling with substance abuse. Holistic treatment approaches should be utilized to address both the SIPD and the craving for substance use, ensuring that patients' mental disorders and substance use issues are treated with equal importance [62, 63].

In pharmacotherapy, high-potency typical antipsychotics have been found effective in reducing psychotic symptoms but insufficient in lowering substance use rates. Conversely, low-potency typical antipsychotics have shown success in reducing substance use rates but are less effective in alleviating psychotic symptoms. Typical antipsychotics are not commonly used in the treatment of SIPD due to their strong dopamine antagonist activity in the mesocorticolimbic reward pathway and their extensive side effect profiles [64].

In the treatment of psychotic disorders induced by PAS, atypical antipsychotics are more commonly preferred due to their ability to target shared neuronal circuits, selectively affect dopamine D2 receptors, positively influence cognitive functions, and modulate serotonin and norepinephrine receptors to improve mood. Additionally, their impact on serotonin 5-hydroxytryptamine 3 (5-HT3) receptors helps reduce the craving for substances. These drugs have also been shown in various studies to reduce obsessive thoughts about substance use through their antiserotonergic effects on 5-HT2 receptors. Furthermore, their antihistaminic mechanisms contribute to sedation, anxiety reduction, and improved sleep [63]. Second-generation antipsychotics that exhibit antagonistic activity at serotonin 5-HT3 receptors have been suggested to reduce substance-seeking behavior [65]. Among the second-generation antipsychotics, *clozapine*, *olanzapine*, and *quetiapine* are the most prominent in the treatment of SIPD [66].

5.1 Psychosocial interventions

5.1.1 Cognitive behavioral therapy in substance-induced psychotic disorder

In SIPD, individuals often have lower motivation for treatment, face difficulties in engaging with therapeutic processes, are more prone to drop out of treatment, and tend to make slower progress. Positive and negative symptoms of psychosis can hinder progress at any stage of treatment. Patients struggling to manage these symptoms may develop unique avoidance strategies and habitualize them as coping mechanisms. Other barriers to personal change include cognitive impairments and diminished social communication skills [67]. Cognitive behavioral therapy (CBT) can be particularly effective in managing psychotic symptoms and reducing substance use. By examining individuals' thoughts, emotions, and behaviors, CBT aims to alter negative thought patterns. It helps develop strategies for managing psychotic symptoms and promoting substance cessation. CBT supports recognizing warning signs and escalating symptoms, managing cravings, finding healthy alternative activities, and using cognitive restructuring to challenge positive beliefs about substance use. This approach fosters greater self-awareness and equips individuals with skills to overcome substance-related challenges [68, 69].

5.1.2 Motivational interviewing

Motivational interviewing focuses on leveraging an individual's strengths and helping them identify the connection between substance use and the challenges it creates in achieving their life goals. A written treatment plan with clear objectives can be developed. The sessions aim to foster coping strategies for avoiding high-risk situations related to substance use and to encourage the development of constructive, substance-free activities [67, 68]. A supportive network of family and friends has been reported to have a significant impact on clinical outcomes and recovery [67].

5.1.3 Group therapies and self-help groups

Group therapies help patients realize they are not alone and that others have experienced similar challenges. In a therapeutic setting, patients can better understand the effects of substance use and psychotic disorders while learning various strategies to cope with substance-induced psychosis. Group therapy also aids in improving interpersonal skills and fostering healthy social relationships. Combining group therapy with pharmacological treatment can enhance the effectiveness of medications and improve patients' adherence to treatment. A study found that individuals who regularly attended group therapy sessions for 1 year or longer demonstrated a reduction in substance use outcomes [70, 71].

Author details

Elif Küçük[1]* and Feride Uysal[2]

1 Department of Psychiatry, Yüksek Ihtisas University, Ankara, Turkey

2 Kartal Dr. Lutfi Kirdar City Hospital, Department of Psychiatry, University of Health Science, Istanbul, Turkey

*Address all correspondence to: drelfkucuk@gmail.com

References

[1] Graham SA, Adamowicz DH, Jeste DV, Lee EE. Schizophrenia Spectrum and Other Psychotic Disorders. Washington, DC, USA: The American Psychiatric Association Publishing Textbook of Geriatric Psychiatry; 2022. p. 311

[2] Mueser KT, Gingerich S. Treatment of co-occurring psychotic and substance use disorders. Social Work in Public Health. 2013;**28**(3-4):424-439. DOI: 10.1080/19371918.2013.774676

[3] Wang Y, Lv J, He J, Wen G, Wu X. Mechanism of psychoactive substance-induced cognitive disorders: Does tau protein play a role? Frontiers in Bioscience (Landmark Edition). 2022;**27**(1):6. DOI: 10.31083/j.fbl2701006

[4] Keshavan MS, Kaneko Y. Secondary psychoses: An update. World Psychiatry. 2013;**12**(1):4-15. DOI: 10.1002/wps.20001

[5] Thirthalli J, Benegal V, Gangdalar BN. Substance-induced psychosis: An overview. In: Keshavan MS, Sachdev PS, editors. Secondary Schizophrenia. Cambridge: Cambridge University Press; 2010. pp. 112-126

[6] Fiorentini A, Cantù F, Crisanti C, Cereda G, Oldani L, Brambilla P. Substance-induced psychoses: An updated literature review. Frontiers in Psychiatry. 2021;**12**:694863. DOI: 10.3389/fpsyt.2021.694863

[7] Pauselli L. Cannabis-induced psychotic disorders. In: Compton MT, Manseau M, editors. The Complex Connection between Cannabis and Schizophrenia. Cambridge, Massachusetts, USA: Academic Press; 2018. pp. 183-197

[8] Köroğlu E. DSM-5 Tanı ölçütleri başvuru el kitabı. Beşinci baskı, Ankara: HYB; 2013

[9] APA. Diagnostic and Statistical Manual of Mental Disorders (DSM-5) 5. 5th ed. Washington, DC, USA: American Psychiatric Association; 2013

[10] World Health Organization. The ICD-10 classification of mental and behavioural disorders: Clinical descriptions and diagnostic guidelines, mental and behavioural disorders due to psychoactive substance use (F10–F19). In: ICD-10 in Psychiatry. Geneva, Switzerland: World Health Organization; 2021

[11] Hjorthøj C, Larsen MO, Starzer MSK, Nordentoft M. Annual incidence of cannabis-induced psychosis, other substance-induced psychoses and dually diagnosed schizophrenia and cannabis use disorder in Denmark from 1994 to 2016. Psychological Medicine. 2021;**51**(4):617-622. DOI: 10.1017/S0033291719003532

[12] Weibell MA, Joa I, Bramness J, et al. Treated incidence and baseline characteristics of substance induced psychosis in a Norwegian catchment area. BMC Psychiatry. 2013;**13**:319. DOI: 10.1186/1471-244X-13-319

[13] Martinotti G, De Risio L, Vannini C, Schifano F, Pettorruso M, Di Giannantonio M. Substance-related exogenous psychosis: A postmodern syndrome. CNS Spectrums. 2021;**26**(1):84-91. DOI: 10.1017/S1092852920001479

[14] Smith MJ, Thirthalli J, Abdallah AB, Murray RM, Cottler LB. Prevalence of psychotic symptoms in substance users: A comparison across substances.

Comprehensive Psychiatry. 2009;**50**(3):245-250. DOI: 10.1016/j.comppsych.2008.07.009

[15] Murray RM, Paparelli A, Morrison PD, Marconi A, Di Forti M. What can we learn about schizophrenia from studying the human model, drug-induced psychosis? American Journal of Medical Genetics. Part B, Neuropsychiatric Genetics. 2013;**162B**(7):661-670. DOI: 10.1002/ajmg.b.32177

[16] Alharbi FF, el-Guebaly N. Cannabis and amphetamine-type stimulant-induced psychoses: A systematic overview. Addictive Disorders & Their Treatment. 2016;**15**(4):190-200

[17] Alderson HL, Semple DM, Blayney C, Queirazza F, Chekuri V, Lawrie SM. Risk of transition to schizophrenia following first admission with substance-induced psychotic disorder: A population-based longitudinal cohort study. Psychological Medicine. 2017;**47**(14):2548-2555. DOI: 10.1017/S0033291717001118

[18] Eseroğlu T, Yalçın Ö, Kılıçoğlu AG, Karaçetin G. The influence of substance use disorder comorbidity on the treatment response of inpatient adolescents with the diagnosis of first episode psychosis. Anadolu Psikiyatri Derg. 2019;**20**(4):385-394. DOI: 10.5455/apd.15238

[19] Montanari L, Guarita B, Mounteney J, Zipfel N, Simon R. Cannabis use among people entering drug treatment in Europe: A growing phenomenon? European Addiction Research. 2017;**23**(3):113-121. DOI: 10.1159/000475810

[20] Rognli EB, Taipale H, Hjorthøj C, et al. Annual incidence of substance-induced psychoses in Scandinavia from 2000 to 2016. Psychological Medicine. 2023;**53**(11):5246-5255. DOI: 10.1017/S003329172200229X

[21] Takakuwa KM, Schears RM. The emergency department care of the cannabis and synthetic cannabinoid patient: A narrative review. International Journal of Emergency Medicine. 2021;**14**(1):10. DOI: 10.1186/s12245-021-00330-3

[22] Seddon JL, Birchwood M, Copello A, et al. Cannabis use is associated with increased psychotic symptoms and poorer psychosocial functioning in first-episode psychosis: A report from the UK national EDEN study. Schizophrenia Bulletin. 2016;**42**(3):619-625. DOI: 10.1093/schbul/sbv154

[23] Fraser S, Hides L, Philips L, Proctor D, Lubman DI. Differentiating first episode substance induced and primary psychotic disorders with concurrent substance use in young people. Schizophrenia Research. 2012;**136**(1-3):110-115. DOI: 10.1016/j.schres.2012.01.022

[24] Mathias S, Lubman DI, Hides L. Substance-induced psychosis: A diagnostic conundrum. The Journal of Clinical Psychiatry. 2008;**69**(3):358-367. DOI: 10.4088/jcp.v69n0304

[25] Schanzer BM, First MB, Dominguez B, Hasin DS, Caton CL. Diagnosing psychotic disorders in the emergency department in the context of substance use. Psychiatric Services. 2006;**57**(10):1468-1473. DOI: 10.1176/ps.2006.57.10.1468

[26] Fennig S, Bromet EJ, Craig T, Jandorf L, Schwartz JE. Psychotic patients with unclear diagnoses. A descriptive analysis. The Journal of Nervous and Mental Disease. 1995;**183**(4):207-213.

DOI: 10.1097/00005053-199504000-00004

[27] Beckmann D, Lowman KL, Nargiso J, McKowen J, Watt L, Yule AM. Substance-induced psychosis in youth. Child and Adolescent Psychiatric Clinics of North America. 2020;**29**(1):131-143. DOI: 10.1016/j.chc.2019.08.006

[28] Boileau I, Dagher A, Leyton M, et al. Modeling sensitization to stimulants in humans: An [11C]raclopride/positron emission tomography study in healthy men. Archives of General Psychiatry. 2006;**63**(12):1386-1395. DOI: 10.1001/archpsyc.63.12.1386

[29] Kim JS, Kornhuber HH, Schmid-Burgk W, Holzmüller B. Low cerebrospinal fluid glutamate in schizophrenic patients and a new hypothesis on schizophrenia. Neuroscience Letters. 1980;**20**(3):379-382. DOI: 10.1016/0304-3940(80)90178-0

[30] Rasmussen H, Erritzoe D, Andersen R, et al. Decreased frontal serotonin2A receptor binding in antipsychotic-naive patients with first-episode schizophrenia. Archives of General Psychiatry. 2010;**67**(1):9-16. DOI: 10.1001/archgenpsychiatry.2009.176

[31] Fiorentini A, Volonteri LS, Dragogna F, et al. Substance-induced psychoses: A critical review of the literature. Current Drug Abuse Reviews. 2011;**4**(4):228-240. DOI: 10.2174/1874473711104040228

[32] Shrivastava A, Johnston M, Terpstra K, Bureau Y. Cannabis and psychosis: Neurobiology. Indian Journal of Psychiatry. 2014;**56**(1):8-16. DOI: 10.4103/0019-5545.124708

[33] Campos AC, Fogaça MV, Sonego AB, Guimarães FS. Cannabidiol, neuroprotection and neuropsychiatric disorders. Pharmacological Research. 2016;**112**:119-127. DOI: 10.1016/j.phrs.2016.01.033

[34] O'Brien K, Blair P. Medicinal Cannabis and CBD in Mental Healthcare. Cham, Switzerland: Springer; 2021

[35] Bloomfield MA, Ashok AH, Volkow ND, Howes OD. The effects of Δ^9-tetrahydrocannabinol on the dopamine system. Nature. 2016;**539**(7629):369-377. DOI: 10.1038/nature20153

[36] Volkow ND, Baler RD, Compton WM, Weiss SR. Adverse health effects of marijuana use. The New England Journal of Medicine. 2014;**370**(23):2219-2227. DOI: 10.1056/NEJMra1402309

[37] Brents LK, Reichard EE, Zimmerman SM, Moran JH, Fantegrossi WE, Prather PL. Phase I hydroxylated metabolites of the K2 synthetic cannabinoid JWH-018 retain in vitro and in vivo cannabinoid 1 receptor affinity and activity. PLoS One. 2011;**6**(7):e21917. DOI: 10.1371/journal.pone.0021917

[38] Fattore L. Synthetic cannabinoids-further evidence supporting the relationship between cannabinoids and psychosis. Biological Psychiatry. 2016;**79**(7):539-548. DOI: 10.1016/j.biopsych.2016.02.001

[39] Sekine Y, Minabe Y, Ouchi Y, et al. Association of dopamine transporter loss in the orbitofrontal and dorsolateral prefrontal cortices with methamphetamine-related psychiatric symptoms. The American Journal of Psychiatry. 2003;**160**(9):1699-1701. DOI: 10.1176/appi.ajp.160.9.1699

[40] Morgan MJ. Ecstasy (MDMA): A review of its possible

persistent psychological effects. Psychopharmacology. 2000;**152**(3):230-248. DOI: 10.1007/s002130000545

[41] Roncero C, Ros-Cucurull E, Daigre C, Casas M. Prevalence and risk factors of psychotic symptoms in cocaine-dependent patients. Actas Españolas de Psiquiatría. 2012;**40**(4):187-197

[42] Parrott AC, Sisk E, Turner JJ. Psychobiological problems in heavy 'ecstasy' (MDMA) polydrug users. Drug and Alcohol Dependence. 2000;**60**(1):105-110. DOI: 10.1016/s0376-8716(99)00146-5

[43] Rognli EB, Bramness JG. Understanding the relationship between amphetamines and psychosis. Current Addiction Reports. 2015;**2**(4):285-292. DOI: 10.1007/s40429-015-0077-4

[44] Henquet C, Krabbendam L, Spauwen J, et al. Prospective cohort study of cannabis use, predisposition for psychosis, and psychotic symptoms in young people. BMJ. 2005;**330**(7481):11. DOI: 10.1136/bmj.38267.664086.63

[45] van Os J, Kenis G, Rutten BP. The environment and schizophrenia. Nature. 2010;**468**(7321):203-212. DOI: 10.1038/nature09563

[46] Veling W. Genetic mediation of the link between schizophrenia and cannabis use. Psychiatry. 2008;**7**(12):511-515. DOI: 10.1016/j.mppsy.2008.10.007

[47] Arunogiri S, McKetin R, Verdejo-Garcia A, Lubman DI. The methamphetamine-associated psychosis spectrum: A clinically focused review. International Journal of Mental Health and Addiction. 2020;**18**(1):54-65. DOI: 10.1007/s11469-018-9934-4

[48] Tang Y, Martin NL, Cotes RO. Cocaine-induced psychotic disorders: Presentation, mechanism, and management. Journal of Dual Diagnosis. 2014;**10**(2):98-105. DOI: 10.1080/15504263.2014.906133

[49] Wilson L, Szigeti A, Kearney A, Clarke M. Clinical characteristics of primary psychotic disorders with concurrent substance abuse and substance-induced psychotic disorders: A systematic review. Schizophrenia Research. 2018;**197**:78-86. DOI: 10.1016/j.schres.2017.11.001

[50] Russo DA, Stochl J, Painter M, et al. Trauma history characteristics associated with mental states at clinical high risk for psychosis. Psychiatry Research. 2014;**220**(1-2):237-244. DOI: 10.1016/j.psychres.2014.08.028

[51] Morrison PD, Zois V, McKeown DA, et al. The acute effects of synthetic intravenous Delta9-tetrahydrocannabinol on psychosis, mood and cognitive functioning. Psychological Medicine. 2009;**39**(10):1607-1616. DOI: 10.1017/S0033291709005522

[52] Tikka SK, D'Souza DC. The association between cannabinoids and psychosis. In: Montoya ID, Weiss SRB, editors. Cannabis Use Disorders. Cham, Switzerland: Springer International Publishing; 2019. pp. 127-155

[53] Winstock AR, Barratt MJ. Synthetic cannabis: A comparison of patterns of use and effect profile with natural cannabis in a large global sample. Drug and Alcohol Dependence. 2013;**131**(1-2):106-111. DOI: 10.1016/j.drugalcdep.2012.12.011

[54] Altintas M, Inanc L, Oruc GA, Arpacioglu S, Gulec H. Clinical characteristics of synthetic cannabinoid-induced psychosis in relation to schizophrenia: A single-center cross-sectional analysis of

concurrently hospitalized patients. Neuropsychiatric Disease and Treatment. 2016;**12**:1893-1900. DOI: 10.2147/NDT.S107622

[55] Rugani F, Bacciardi S, Rovai L, et al. Symptomatological features of patients with and without ecstasy use during their first psychotic episode. International Journal of Environmental Research and Public Health. 2012;**9**(7):2283-2292. DOI: 10.3390/ijerph9072283

[56] McGuire PK, Cope H, Fahy TA. Diversity of psychopathology associated with use of 3,4-methylene-dioxymethamphetamine ('Ecstasy'). The British Journal of Psychiatry. 1994;**165**(3):391-395. DOI: 10.1192/bjp.165.3.391

[57] Janowsky DS, Risch C. Amphetamine psychosis and psychotic symptoms. Psychopharmacology. 1979;**65**(1):73-77. DOI: 10.1007/BF00491982

[58] Voce A, Calabria B, Burns R, Castle D, McKetin R. A systematic review of the symptom profile and course of methamphetamine-associated psychosis substance use and misuse. Substance Use & Misuse. 2019;**54**(4):549-559. DOI: 10.1080/10826084.2018.1521430

[59] Wearne TA, Cornish JL. A comparison of methamphetamine-induced psychosis and schizophrenia: A review of positive, negative, and cognitive symptomatology. Frontiers in Psychiatry. 2018;**9**:491. DOI: 10.3389/fpsyt.2018.00491

[60] Caton CL, Samet S, Hasin DS. When acute-stage psychosis and substance use co-occur: Differentiating substance-induced and primary psychotic disorders. Journal of Psychiatric Practice. 2000;**6**(5):256-266. DOI: 10.1097/00131746-200009000-00006

[61] Serper MR, Chou JC, Allen MH, Czobor P, Cancro R. Symptomatic overlap of cocaine intoxication and acute schizophrenia at emergency presentation. Schizophrenia Bulletin. 1999;**25**(2):387-394. DOI: 10.1093/oxfordjournals.schbul.a033386

[62] Green AI, Zimmet SV, Strous RD, Schildkraut JJ. Clozapine for comorbid substance use disorder and schizophrenia: Do patients with schizophrenia have a reward-deficiency syndrome that can be ameliorated by clozapine? Harvard Review of Psychiatry. 1999;**6**(6):287-296. DOI: 10.3109/10673229909017206

[63] Karaoğlan M, Kaşarcı G, Şahin E, İplik ES. Atypical antipsychotics in the treatment of substance-related psychotic disorders. Experimed. 2020;**10**(1):49-58. DOI: 10.26650/experimed.2020.0005

[64] McEvoy JP, Freudenreich O, Levin ED, Rose JE. Haloperidol increases smoking in patients with schizophrenia. Psychopharmacology. 1995;**119**(1):124-126. DOI: 10.1007/BF02246063

[65] Bymaster FP, Falcone JF, Bauzon D, et al. Potent antagonism of 5-HT(3) and 5-HT(6) receptors by olanzapine. European Journal of Pharmacology. 2001;**430**(2-3):341-349. DOI: 10.1016/s0014-2999(01)01399-1

[66] Akerman SC, Brunette MF, Noordsy DL, Green AI. Pharmacotherapy of co-occurring schizophrenia and substance use disorders. Current Addiction Reports. 2014;**1**(4):251-260. DOI: 10.1007/s40429-014-0034-7

[67] Mueser KT, Drake RE, Sigmon SC, Brunette MF. Psychosocial interventions for adults with severe mental illnesses and co-occurring substance use disorders. Journal of Dual Diagnosis.

2005;**1**:57-82. DOI: 10.1300/J374v01n02_05

[68] Kavanagh DJ, Young R, White A, et al. A brief motivational intervention for substance misuse in recent-onset psychosis. Drug and Alcohol Review. 2004;**23**(2):151-155. DOI: 10.1080/09595230410001704127

[69] Baker A, Bucci S, Lewin TJ, Kay-Lambkin F, Constable PM, Carr VJ. Cognitive-behavioural therapy for substance use disorders in people with psychotic disorders: Randomised controlled trial. The British Journal of Psychiatry. 2006;**188**:439-448. DOI: 10.1192/bjp.188.5.439

[70] Horsfall J, Cleary M, Hunt GE, Walter G. Psychosocial treatments for people with co-occurring severe mental illnesses and substance use disorders (dual diagnosis): A review of empirical evidence. Harvard Review of Psychiatry. 2009;**17**(1):24-34. DOI: 10.1080/10673220902724599

[71] Mortan Sevi O, Tekinsav SS. Şizofreni ve diğer psikotik bozukluklarda bilişsel-davranışçı grup terapisi-sistematik bir gözden geçirme [Cognitive-behavioral group treatment for schizophrenia and other psychotic disorders - A systematic review]. Türk Psikiyatri Dergisi. 2012;**23**(3):206-218

Chapter 7

Treatment of Hypomania

Mustafa Akkuş

Abstract

Hypomania is a mood period that is often described by patients as a more energetic and desired period. However, unfortunately, it is sometimes ignored by relatives of the patient because its symptoms are not very severe. It can also be a significant problem for clinicians since it is not easily recognized by them or they do not have enough knowledge about its treatment. Hypomania is generally considered as mild or short-lasting mania, in the ICD and DSM classification systems, it is defined differently, and clinicians display different approaches toward it. In the treatment of hypomania, both pharmacological and non-pharmacological methods are used. In the pharmacological approach, some antipsychotics and mood stabilizing drugs are administered. In addition to medication therapy, implementation of non-pharmacological methods such as interpersonal and social rhythm therapy, behavioral therapy, cognitive therapy, and some psychoeducational interventions is also effective in this period.

Keywords: hypomania, bipolar II disorder, pharmacological treatment, psychotherapy, mood

1. Introduction

Hypomania is a milder form of mania, during which the person feels extremely happy, more energetic and powerful than usual, and more productive. The symptoms can be noticed by patients and their relatives, but they may not be as life disrupting as they are in mania. People are mostly happy during this period and may not be able to foresee risky situations and may stop using their medications.

In some cases, hypomania diagnosis can be missed. There are clinical difficulties in the diagnosis and evaluation of hypomania. Therefore, as studies on the diagnosis and treatment of hypomania increase, this period will be better understood. In this chapter of the book, it was aimed to evaluate the diagnosis and differential diagnosis of hypomania and to discuss the pharmacological and non-pharmacological treatment approaches in the treatment of hypomania in line with the current literature.

2. Method

While this chapter of the book was written, PubMed and Google academic databases were scanned, studies on the diagnostic evaluation and treatment approaches of hypomania, and treatment guidelines were reviewed, a large number of studies were scanned within this context, and the chapter was prepared by citing 14 studies.

The inclusion criteria for this chapter of the book were as follows: being treatment guidelines, being books with an important place in the literature, being publications with a higher number of citations, and being publications that will add new and interesting information to the literature on the subject. Case reports and publications with a relatively lower level of evidence were not included in this chapter of the book.

3. Hypomania diagnoses and differential diagnoses

According to the ICD-10, hypomania corresponds to mild mania and does not include a duration criterion. According to the DSM-5, hypomania is defined as a period of elevated mood that requires at least four days. The distinction between mania and hypomania is one of the most controversial points of classification systems. DSM makes this distinction in terms of severity and duration. Hypomania is defined as a clinical picture that lasts at least 4 days, does not require hospitalization, does not have a traumatic effect on the person's life, and does not have psychotic symptoms; however, the change in mood and functional level is noticed by others. Reliability and therefore validity of hypomania diagnosis is low, in terms of both its duration and its difference from ordinary mood swings or mild mania. ICD-10, which distinguishes mania from hypomania as a difference in severity, is more understandable in this respect. [1]

According to DSM-5, the diagnostic criteria for hypomania are as follows:

- It is an elevated, grandiose, or irritable mood that is markedly different from usual mood and lasts at least 4 days
- Presence of at least three (or four if mood is irritable) of the following symptoms during the mood episode:
  - o Increased self-esteem, grandiosity
  - o Decreased need for sleep
  - o Being overly talkative, pressured speech
  - o Flight of ideas
  - o Distraction
  - o Psychomotor agitation, increased goal-directed activities
  - o Participating in pleasurable activities whose probability of producing negative consequences is high
  - o It is not due to the effects of a substance or general medical condition.

There is continuing interest in cases on the spectrum with less severe mood elevations as an extension of the bipolar diagnosis.

Bipolar disorder not otherwise specified (NOS), a DSM-IV diagnosis, includes any of the following: (1) recurrent subthreshold hypomania in the presence of intercurrent major depression, (2) recurrent hypomania (at least two episodes) in the absence of recurrent major depression, and the presence or absence of subthreshold major depression, and (3) recurrent subthreshold hypomania in the absence of intercurrent major depression, and in the presence or absence of subthreshold major depression.

The number of symptoms essential to diagnose subthreshold hypomania is two of the B symptoms (three required for DSM-IV, or four if mood is irritable). DSM-5 changed the diagnosis of 'bipolar NOS' to 'other specified bipolar and related disorder'; however, this still covers the same group of disorders. The lifetime incidence of these disorders in the population is 2.4% [2].

On the other hand, Akiskal classified bipolar disorder as follows and specified hypomania in more than one group.

- BP-½ SchizoBP
- BP-I Mania
- BP-I½ Prolonged hypomanic depression
- BP-II Spontaneous hypomanic depression
- BP-II½ Cyclothymic depressions
- BP-III Hypomania with AD
- BP-III½ Masked BP with stimulant use
- BP-IV Hyperthymic depression [3].

Hypomania screening assessment is performed using the Hypomania Checklist-32 Renewed Version (HCL-32-R).

Hypomania Checklist –32 Renewed Version (HCL-32-R):

- It is a self-report scale.
- Its first two items are rated on a Likert-type scale.
- It measures general mood and energy/activity level.
- Its third item consists of 32 statements answered as yes/no.
- Its cut-off score is 14 (70% specificity-sensitivity was determined).
- It contains different dimensions.
- It assesses exuberance/increased energy.
- It assesses risky behaviors/impulsivity [4].

4. Treatment of hypomania

Bipolar II disorder is a group of bipolar disorders in which major depression and hypomania episodes are observed. Hypomania is treated by providing treatment during the episode and preventive treatment to prevent hypomania from occurring. Pharmacotherapy of hypomania is presented in **Table 1**.

4.1 Acute treatment of hypomania

General principles of mania treatment are also applied in the treatment of hypomania. In some patients, hypomania causes minimal or no impairment in functioning and may even lead to functioning above normal for short periods. On the other hand, prolonged, relatively severe, mixed, or irritable hypomania may impair functioning. Treatment of hypomania includes not only discontinuation of medications such as antidepressants and stimulants that may prolong the duration of symptoms or worsen symptoms but also initiation of appropriate pharmacotherapy. Unfortunately, whether many standard medications used for mania such as lithium and atypical antipsychotics could be used for hypomania has not been adequately studied.

The following four placebo-controlled drug studies have been conducted on acute hypomania: divalproex (level 4), N-acetylcysteine (level 4), quetiapine (level 4), and one open-label study of risperidone (level 4). In these studies, the focus is generally on efficacy. Although all these studies had significant weaknesses, some included small sample sizes, and some included samples with diagnoses of bipolar I disorder, bipolar II disorder, bipolar disorder not otherwise specified, and diagnoses of hypomania and mania. Positive results were obtained not in all but in some of them.

4.2 Maintenance treatment of hypomania

In different guidelines, different recommendations are made to treat hypomania. Recommended treatments for maintenance treatment of bipolar II disorder by level of evidence are as follows:

First line treatments:

- Quetiapine-Level 1
- Lithium-Level 2
- Lamotrigine-Level 2

Acute treatment of hypomania	Maintenance treatment of (Bipolar II)-hypomania-
Discontinuation of medications such as antidepressants and stimulants	Quetiapine
Divalproex	Lithium
N-acetylcysteine	Carbamazepine
Quetiapine	Divalproex
Risperidone	Risperidone(primarily hypomania prevention)

Table 1.
Pharmacological treatment of hypomania.

- Second line treatment:
- Venlafaxine-Level 2
- Third line treatments:
- Carbamazepine-Level 3
- Sodium valproate-Level 3
- Escitalopram-Level 3
- Fluoxetine- Level 3
- Other antidepressants-Level 3
- Fourth line treatment

Risperidone-level 4

In the treatment of bipolar II disorder, while risperidone is effective primarily for the prevention of hypomania, other medications are effective primarily for the prevention of depression [5].

Some general recommendations on the treatment of hypomania are as follows:

- Patients in the hypomanic period should be enabled to access calming environments and reduced stimuli.
- They should be advised not to make important decisions until they come out of the hypomanic period, and, if possible, they should be encouraged to maintain their relationships with their relatives.
- If a person using antidepressants develops hypomania, the antidepressant should be discontinued, and an appropriate antipsychotic should be prescribed.
- If a person who has not taken any mood stabilizer or antipsychotic medication develops mania or hypomania, it is recommended to prescribe haloperidol, olanzapine, quetiapine, or risperidone as antipsychotics, by taking previous preconceptions, the person's preference, and clinical characteristics (physical comorbidity, previous treatment response, and side effects) into account.
- If the first antipsychotic taken by the person is not well tolerated at any dose (due to reasons such as rapid weight gain) or is not effective at the maximum licensed dose, it is recommended to switch to an alternative antipsychotic from the recommended list above.
- If one of the alternative antipsychotics is not effective enough at the maximum licensed doses, it should be considered to add lithium to the treatment. If the addition of lithium is not effective or if lithium treatment is not suitable for the individual (e.g., if the individual does not accept routine blood monitoring), it

should be considered to add valproate to the treatment. Valproate should not be recommended to women or girls of childbearing potential. Valproate should not be chosen for acute attack treatment or long-term treatment unless other treatment options are inadequate or tolerable.

- If a person using an antidepressant and a mood stabilizer together develops mania or hypomania, the antidepressant should be discontinued.

- If the person is already taking lithium, plasma lithium levels should be checked to ensure the effectiveness of the treatment, and it should be considered to add haloperidol, olanzapine, quetiapine or risperidone to the treatment, considering the person's preference and response to previous treatment.

- If the person is taking valproate or another mood stabilizer as a preventive measure, it should be considered to increase the dose and the dose should be increased to the maximum effective dose depending on the clinical response. If there is no improvement, one of the antipsychotics (haloperidol, olanzapine, quetiapine, or risperidone) should be added, taking into account the person's preference and previous treatment response. If a woman or girl of childbearing potential is already taking valproate, she should be informed that any exposure to valproate during pregnancy can cause fetal malformations and adverse neurodevelopmental outcomes and that the drug should be slowly tapered off and then discontinued.

- If the clinical manifestation is a mixed affective state consisting of manic and depressive symptoms, the aforementioned recommendations to prevent hypomania should be fulfilled, and the patient should be closely monitored for depressive states.

- Lamotrigine is not recommended for the treatment of mania [6].

5. The role of psychotherapy

The number of studies conducted on the effectiveness of psychotherapy for bipolar II disorder is rather limited, and the number of studies directly measuring the effects of these treatments on hypomania is even fewer. In psychotherapies, attention is paid to mood cycles and recognition of these cycles, traumas associated with the

Cognitive therapy
Cognitive–behavioral therapy
Psychoeducation
Family-focused therapy
Case management
Interpersonal social rhythm therapy

Table 2.
Nonpharmacological treatment of hypomania.

illness can be targeted, and the psychosocial outcomes of the illness can be improved. It is unlikely to observe the monotherapy effect of psychotherapy in studies because patients receive psychotherapy as an adjunctive therapy while they use psychiatric medications. Among psychotherapy methods whose effectiveness has been proven are cognitive therapy, cognitive–behavioral therapy, psychoeducation, family-focused therapy, case management, and interpersonal social rhythm therapy [7]. These methods are presented in **Table 2**.

6. Role of interpersonal and social rhythm therapy

Preliminary evidence for the effectiveness of interpersonal and social rhythm therapy (IPSRT) in bipolar II disorder has been demonstrated [8]. IPSRT is the only psychotherapy which indicates that it is possible to treat individuals with bipolar II disorder with psychotherapy alone [9]. IPSRT is based on an instability model that identifies three interconnected pathways leading to relapse. These pathways are stressful life events, medication non-compliance, and social rhythm disruption. In addition, in this therapy, theories about the role of social and environmental cues in maintaining circadian rhythm integrity are gaining importance. In this theory, social cues that form the routine disrupt the sleep–wake cycle, which can lead to disruptions in mood such as hypomania, depression, etc. IPSRT comprises three main sections: psychoeducation, social rhythm therapy, and interpersonal relationships.

Therapists particularly draw attention to the history of rhythm disturbances, especially sleep disturbances, preceding the attacks.

It is often rather difficult to persuade individuals with bipolar II disorder to make significant changes in their daily routine such as going to bed at the same time every day, because initially, there is little apparent reason to make these changes. Effects of these changes in preventing hypomania are uncertain, because patients may perceive hypomania as a relief from depression and may not welcome this treatment proposal because hypomania is not accompanied by the negative consequences associated with mania. Individuals with bipolar II may have less insight into their symptoms than do those with bipolar I, and they may not recognize the symptoms of hypomania [10]. In order to encourage rhythm regulation, it should be emphasized that a period of depression may be followed by a period of hypomania and that the goal of this therapy is to improve general mood stability. Patients should be asked to reconsider that benign nature of hypomania, which is not as destructive as some patients think, and to view it as a kind of 'experiment' to see whether it is beneficial to general mood, energy, and motivation. If patients can observe the change in their mood when they fail to maintain a regular schedule, they may be more successful in maintaining rhythm stability.

Because of the subtlety of hypomania and the complexity of the mixed states, it may be difficult to assess the mood of individuals with bipolar II disorder accurately. Therefore, therapeutic gains may also be difficult. Assessing energy change rather than mood may be easier in following these patients [11].

Patients are taught to adjust the level of stimulation in their lives according to their mood, to increase stimulation when their mood is low and to decrease stimulation when they are vulnerable to hypomania. Some patients will paradoxically create chaos in their lives when they feel better, because euthymic mood is often experienced as 'flat'. Hypomanic mood may motivate these individuals to make choices that further elevate their mood without being aware that their choices have the potential to lead to interpersonal chaos or more serious mood changes. Therefore, therapists should teach their patients to recognize the negative aspects of participating in stimulating activities and to identify appropriate activities that regulate stimulation.

Grandiosity and entitlement levels of individuals with bipolar II disorder may be high [12]. Although grandiosity is a symptom of hypomania, the individual may have high levels of grandiosity at baseline, regardless of mood. Most patients are open to having these behaviors pointed out by a supportive therapist with whom they have a close therapeutic relationship. Therapists are likely to be faced with maladaptive interpersonal patterns while they establish a therapeutic relationship; thus, they must know how to recognize, tolerate, and manage these difficulties.

Individuals with mixed moods display high levels of emotional reactivity, which can lead to difficulty downregulating arousal levels even when they are not in an acute mood episode. Therefore, therapists may benefit from other helpful strategies such as breathing exercises, distraction, and self-soothing to reduce the rapid shifting of emotions.

Patients should be asked if they use legal and illegal drugs and alcohol and should be informed about the effects of these substances on mood. Among these substances, most common ones are alcohol, prescription drugs, street drugs, nicotine, and caffeine. Caffeine can increase energy in people who are generally low in energy, so caution should be taken as it can cause hypomanic symptoms.

IPSRT can be used in combination with medication used in bipolar II disorder and may be useful in preventing hypomania and other episodes. It is also clear that more experience with psychotherapy is required [13].

7. Cognitive interventions in hypomanic episode

During a hypomanic episode, the person may have unrealistic positive beliefs such as 'I am better than everyone else,' 'I can do whatever I want,' or 'I will be strong and energetic from now on' about themselves, the world, and the future. In addition, he or she may have such beliefs that the illness can pass by his or her own will or that there is no need for medication. It is attempted to regulate cognition by targeting beliefs and cognitive distortions related to this.

8. Behavioral interventions in hypomanic episode

Activity programming can also be effectively achieved during the hypomanic period. Behavioral patterns in this period differ from those in the depressive period. It may be beneficial to reduce the activities that are rewarding for the person in hypomania. The following behavioral suggestions are also useful:

- Increasing the amount of sleep: A decrease in the amount of sleep is a symptom of hypomania and affects the elevation in mood. The aim is to ensure that the person sleeps more than they think is sufficient, close to the amount of sleep they have in the euthymic period. Activities such as going out at night and participating in night entertainment that delay going to sleep should be restricted in the program.

- Tightening money management: Monthly and weekly budget arrangements can be made in cooperation with the patient. Taking measures to limit the person's access to financial sources may be useful. Limiting shopping expenses above a certain limit may be useful. Restrictive measures can be taken on bank accounts. For the effectiveness of these periods, communication with the patient should be continued during the hypomanic period. Interventions should be repeated in each attack.

- Slowing down the making of important decisions: It is recommended that the patient should make decisions likely to create major material and spiritual changes in his or her life only after two consecutive nights of adequate sleep. It is also recommended that decisions should be made after at least two reliable people are counseled before any decision is made. When this approach is explained to the patient, the decision-making mechanism of large companies or the referee system in scientific research can be given as examples.

- Reducing impulsive behaviors: A person in an elevated mood is advised to think for five seconds before he or she takes an action while arguing or joking with others and to visualize two different outcomes of this action. For example, in response to a dirty joke, they are asked to imagine the other person smiling or distressed.

- Stimulus regulation: The aim is to avoid stimuli that may be associated with elevated mood or dysphoria in the person's activity program. These stimuli may be specific places, people, or conditions or may be related to a specific friend, or they may be focused on a specific area such as writing an article, or physiological states such as hunger or fatigue [14].

9. Conclusion

In the present study, it was aimed to ensure the correct recognition of hypomania, which is a mood episode that is often overlooked by researchers and clinicians, and to present pharmacological and nonpharmacological treatment approaches. It is thought that this chapter is important because it is expected to provide guidance to future studies in the field of hypomania.

Author details

Mustafa Akkuş
Erzincan Binali Yıldırım University, Erzincan, Turkey

*Address all correspondence to: drmustafaakkus@gmail.com

References

[1] Parker G, Fletcher K. Differentiating bipolar I and II disorders and the likely contribution of DSM-V classification to their cleavage. Journal of Affective Disorders. 2014;**152**:154-157. DOI: 10.1016/j.jad.2013.10.006

[2] Goodwin GM, Haddad PM, Ferrier IN, Aronson JK, Barnes T, Cipriani A, et al. Evidence-based guidelines for treating bipolar disorder: Revised third edition recommendations from the British Association for Psychopharmacology. Journal of Psychopharmacology. 2016;**30**:495-553. DOI: 10.1177/0269881116636545

[3] Akiskal HS, Pinto O. The evolving bipolar spectrum. Prototypes I, II, III, and IV. The Psychiatric Clinics of North America. 1999;**22**:517-534. DOI: 10.1016/s0193-953x(05)70093-9

[4] Vahip S, Aydemir O, Akkaya C, Altınbaş K, Kora K, Suculluoglu Dikici D, et al. Türk Psikiyatri Dergisi. 2017;**28**: 117-123

[5] Yatham LN, Kennedy SH, Parikh SV, Schaffer A, Bond DJ, Frey BN, et al. Canadian network for mood and anxiety treatments (CANMAT) and International Society for Bipolar Disorders (ISBD) 2018 guidelines for the management of patients with bipolar disorder. Bipolar Disorders. 2018;**20**:97-170. DOI: 10.1111/bdi.12609

[6] Kendall T, Morriss R, Mayo-Wilson E, Marcus E. Guideline development Group of the National Institute for health and care excellence. Assessment and management of bipolar disorder: summary of updated NICE guidance. BMJ. 2014;**349**:g5673. DOI: 10.1136/bmj.g5673

[7] Novick DM, Swartz HA. Psychosocial interventions for bipolar II disorder. American Journal of Psychotherapy. 2019;**72**:47-57. DOI: 10.1176/appi.psychotherapy.20190008

[8] Miklowitz DJ, Otto MW, Frank E, Reilly-Harrington NA, Wisniewski SR, Kogan JN, et al. Psychosocial treatments for bipolar depression: a 1-year randomized trial from the Systematic Treatment Enhancement Program. Archives of General Psychiatry. 2007;**64**:419-426. DOI: 10.1001/archpsyc.64.4.419

[9] Swartz HA, Frank E, Frankel DR, Novick D, Houck P. Psychotherapy as monotherapy for the treatment of bipolar II depression: A proof of concept study. Bipolar Disorders. 2009;**11**:89-94. DOI: 10.1111/j.1399-5618.2008.00629.x

[10] Pallanti S, Quercioli L, Pazzagli A, Rossi A, Dell'Osso L, Pini S, et al. Awareness of illness and subjective experience of cognitive complaints in patients with bipolar I and bipolar II disorder. The American Journal of Psychiatry. 1999;**156**:1094-1096. DOI: 10.1176/ajp.156.7.1094

[11] Koukopoulos A. Ewald Hecker's description of cyclothymia as a cyclical mood disorder: its relevance to the modern concept of bipolar II. Journal of Affective Disorders. 2003;**73**:199-205. DOI: 10.1016/s0165-0327(02)00326-9

[12] Gartner JD. The Hypomanic Edge: The Link between a Little Craziness and a Lot of Success in America. New York: Simon and Schuster; 2005

[13] Swartz HA, Levenson JC, Frank E. Psychotherapy for bipolar II disorder: The role of interpersonal and social

rhythm therapy. Professional Psychology: Research and Practice. 2012;**43**:145-153. DOI: 10.1037/a0027671

[14] Ozdel K, Kart A, Turkcapar MH. Cognitive Behavioral Therapy in Treatment of Bipolar Disorder. Noro Psikiyatri Arsivi. 2021;**58**:66-76. DOI: 10.29399/npa.27419

Section 4

Technology and Societal Impacts

Chapter 8

Mental Health Prediction Model in Eswatini Using Machine Learning Techniques

Stephen Fashoto, Ndumiso Ginindza, Sibusiso Dlamini and Olubunmi Fashoto

Abstract

Mental health is a very important aspect of our daily life because it includes our emotional, psychological, and social well-being. It affects how we think, feel, and act. Mental and physical health are equally important components of overall health. Depression increases the risk for many types of physical health problems, particularly long-lasting conditions like diabetes, heart disease, and stroke. Similarly, the presence of chronic conditions can increase the risk of mental illness. In this study, we performed an analysis on the Eswatini Ministry of Health Dataset and discovered interesting patterns on mental health in the Kingdom of Eswatini. A machine learning models were developed for predicting anxiety and depression using the given features in the dataset. From this, a conclusion was drawn after comparing the findings from this study with the existing literature from an international perspective on predicting anxiety and depression. The models are compared based on their ability to train with the lowest error values. Streamlit was used to build the application that runs the model. This study concludes that early detection, such as identifying individuals at risk of developing anxiety or depression, can enable early intervention and prevent the progression of symptoms.

Keywords: mental health, anxiety, depression, machine learning, CRISP-ML(Q), Eswatini

1. Introduction

The incidence of mental illness globally and in Eswatini is increasing at an alarming rate. The coronavirus (Covid-19) pandemic exacerbated mental health illness among the populace due to lockdown and restriction of movement. Due to the increase in the occurrence and global burden of mental illnesses, the prevention and treatment of mental health disorders have become a public health priority [1]. Early detection of mental illness enables mental healthcare professionals to treat and enhance the patient's well-being. According to Thieme [1], mental health disorders may lead to suicide. A report on a population survey of persons aged 15–69 years in Eswatini showed that one in ten participants had engaged in suicidal ideation, plans, and/or attempts in the past

12 months, and 3.6% had attempted suicide [2]. The high prevalence of mental illness and the need for effective mental health care, combined with recent advances in Artificial Intelligence (AI), have led to an increase in explorations of how the field of machine learning (ML) can assist in the detection, diagnosis, and treatment of mental health problems [1]. The role of digital technology in improving healthcare has increased significantly and has led to a variety of health technologies and applications. To explore this area, there is a need for the availability of relevant datasets. There has been growth in data availability for mental health worldwide, and Eswatini has followed suit after the establishment of the Health Management Information System (HMIS).

In the past, mental health disorder relied on traditional approaches that were constructed from expert opinion and classified according to the International Classification of Diseases (ICD). Currently, instead of the conventional approach, statistical, machine learning, natural language processing techniques, and neuroimaging have been investigated for prompt detection of persistent depressive disorder (PDD) [3–5]; however, the dependability of such findings is ambiguous as a result of methodological approaches that could have been exaggerated in previous literature. Further, two key drawbacks exist in the literatures that hamper the translational applicability in actual clinical practice [6]. The application of machine learning-based diagnostic tools for the detection of mental health illness [6] for clinical-based practices contrasts with actual practice because early diagnosis of mental health disorders could be complicated. Diagnosing persistent depressive disorder in an individual could be nerve-racking [7], but mental healthcare professionals require the medical and psychiatric background of patients to aid clinical assessment.

In Eswatini, mental illness is a threat, and the need for mental health services is extremely high. Small-scale studies attest to the fact that common mental disorders such as depression, anxiety, and substance use are highly prevalent in the population of Eswatini [8]. What is more fascinating is that individuals may not display symptoms until it is too late. Another challenge is the service organization of mental health; there is no mental health unit dedicated to the coordination of mental health services in the Kingdom of Eswatini. Consequently, services for mental health in Eswatini are not well coordinated, integrated, or decentralized. Furthermore, there are minimal mental health promotion and prevention initiatives in the kingdom. There is a lack of appropriate measures to increase awareness and sensitization of individuals, communities, and vulnerable and special at-risk groups on mental health [8].

According to the Ministry of Health (MOH) National Mental Health Strategic and Implementation Plan 2020–2025, mental health services are not fully decentralized in the country; nurse-led services are provided at primary and secondary levels of health care. Comprehensive inpatient and outpatient mental health services are only delivered at tertiary care, which is the National Psychiatric Referral Hospital. This is despite strong evidence that the majority of the uncomplicated Common Mental Disorders (CMD) burden could be treated by non-specialists in the community without sophisticated medical technology.

In Eswatini, there is a lack of capacity and strategy to deliver basic standardized mental health interventions for early detection and treatment, particularly at primary and secondary levels of care. The Kingdom of Eswatini has a national essential drug list in line with WHO recommendations that comprises psychiatric medicines; however, there is a limited supply of psychiatric medicines at all levels of care. Consequently, there is a large burden of preventable mental illness in the kingdom.

Another shortfall of mental health in Eswatini is data and evidence. Population-level burden, process, and outcome data to support the closure of the treatment gap

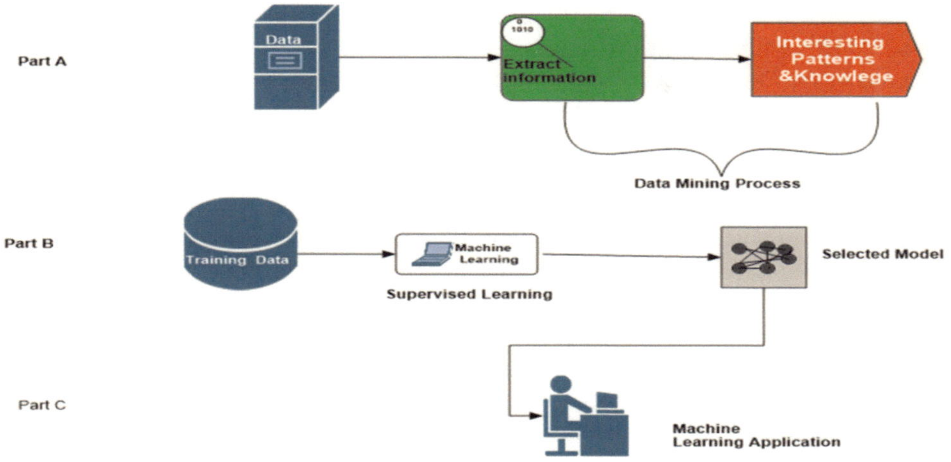

Figure 1.
The concept of the study.

are severely lacking. The National Healthcare Management Information System provides limited access to the Client Management Information System (CMIS). There is also limited research and funding dedicated to mental health in the Kingdom of Eswatini. The scarcity of data on the true burden, distribution, and outcomes of CMD inhibits the efficient use of limited resources that are available for mental health services. Furthermore, in the absence of robust clinical and epidemiological evidence, the investment case for mental health is weak, particularly in light of more visible, better-monitored health conditions such as HIV, TB, and maternal health.

The study aims to apply machine learning models to predict depression and anxiety illnesses in Eswatini using the dataset from the Health Management Information System (HMIS), as shown in **Figure 1**.

2. Literature review

The World Health Organization (WHO) has defined "mental health" as the condition of a person who is able to handle his/her stress in life according to his/her ability but is still able to work normally and productively as well as contribute to the society [9]. Mental disorders present a global health concern, while the diagnosis of mental disorders can be challenging [10]. The diagnosis is even harder for patients who have more than one type of mental disorder, especially for young toddlers who are required to complete questionnaires or standardized rating scales for diagnosis [10]. Mental illnesses, such as depression, are highly prevalent and have been shown to impact an individual's physical health [11]. A technical revolution in mental health care is approaching [12]. The timely identification of patients who are at risk of a mental health crisis can lead to improved outcomes and mitigate burdens and costs [13]. However, a psychiatric clinical examination consists of an interview regarding the past and present symptoms and observing the current pathological signs. The mental status exam (MSE) is a standardized form of examination with methods for observing and describing the mental state and behaviors of each patient, based on both objective observations of the clinician and subjective descriptions given by the patient [14].

According to [9], more than 400 million people worldwide are affected by mental illness, which is almost half the number of people who have diabetes globally. Over 100 million are living with mental illness in Africa, as reported by the World Health Organization in 2022. In Africa, the burden of mental health is rising rapidly, yet critical questions about its prevalence and causes remain unanswered due to limited data.

The World Health Organization (WHO) estimated that one in four individuals' experiences mental disorders at any stage of their lives [9]. The current changes in the social landscape have contributed significantly to the increase in the rate of mental health problems and psychological disorders [9]. The high prevalence of mental illness and the need for effective mental health care, combined with recent advances in AI, have led to an increase in explorations of how the field of machine learning (ML) can assist in the detection, diagnosis, and treatment of mental health problems [1].

According to Ref. [15], mental health problems are based on biological factors as well as social and socioeconomic environments. The main factors leading to mental health problems among higher education students are lack of social support, financial troubles, and the learning environment. The lack of social support is defined as insufficient support within the community that ultimately increases stress. The support from family members and other people around a student can positively impact them. Otherwise, the student is bound to experience loneliness, hence increasing their stress level, which may lead to mental health problems such as depression and anxiety disorders. Biological factors in mental health problems refer to the abnormal functioning of nerve cell circuits or pathways that connect the brain regions, which may be caused by genetics, infection due to brain damage, brain defect, or prenatal damage, among other factors. Social environment refers to how a person interacts with their surroundings, culture, or way of life. It is about the person's relationship with their family, friends, colleagues, and local community, the lack of social support, and discrimination at the workplace. The socio-economic environment reflects the person's financial status. Financial difficulty can become a major factor that causes mental health problems, as people with low financial standing are prone to stress and anxiety. Learning environment refers to daily life at university, assessments, and learning styles.

Mental health is increasingly acknowledged as an important public health concern in Eswatini. Mental disorders are highly prevalent and cause significant suffering, and the disease burden is high. According to the National Mental Health Strategic and Implementation Plan 2020–2025, population-level data is scarce in the country, and therefore, there is a need for comprehensive, integrated, and well-coordinated mental health services in Eswatini. In the strategic plan, it is also mentioned that the treatment gap for mental health disorders in the Kingdom of Eswatini is large, though it varies across the four regions (Manzini, Hhohho, Lubombo, and Shiselweni). There is only one health facility in the Manzini region, the National Psychiatric Referral Hospital (NPRH), that delivers specialized inpatient and outpatient psychiatric care for 1.1 million EmaSwati citizens, with only one resident psychiatrist working to meet the advanced psychiatric needs of the entire kingdom. It is estimated that one in ten EmaSwati adults have seriously considered suicide, and only a quarter of these report seeking professional help. One of the priority interventions of the Ministry of Health (MOH) is to strengthen information systems, evidence, and research for mental health by developing and incorporating mental health indicators into the Healthcare Management Information Systems (HMIS). This is envisaged to promote research priorities for mental health and facilitate knowledge translation on conducted mental health research to guide decision-making.

Machine learning techniques are currently popular approaches for mental health problem detection [9]. Previous research used classification techniques to detect many types of mental health problems, such as stress, suicidal ideation, distress, and depression [9]. The high prevalence of mental illness combined with the need for effective health care has led to an increase in the investigation of how machine learning can assist in the detection and diagnosis of mental health problems. Machine learning techniques can potentially offer new routes for learning patterns of human behavior; identifying mental health symptoms and risk factors; developing predictions about disease progression; and personalizing and optimizing therapies [1].

Machine learning is a data-driven technology that can learn from past data and automatically improve, can detect various patterns in data from the given dataset, and is similar to data mining because it also deals with a huge amount of data. Machine learning can be divided into four categories: supervised learning, unsupervised learning, semi-supervised learning, and reinforcement learning. The best models with the highest accuracy are the decision tree for stress and the support vector machine for depression. Linear regression and neural networks are the two models that gave fair results for anxiety, with an accuracy range between 68% and 88% for the research on predicting mental illness in Malaysia [15].

When examining recent research in computing and HCI addressing machine learning in mental health, it covers the detection and diagnosis of mental health symptoms or conditions, prediction of mental health risks, and understanding of mental health-related behaviors [1]. This has happened at the global level, but when it comes to the local domain, no machine learning has been done on the available data.

3. Methodology

The methodology guide for undertaking this study is the use of the Cross-Industry Standard Process for the development of Machine Learning applications with Quality Assurance (CRISP-ML(Q)). For each phase of the process model as presented in **Figure 2**, the quality assurance approach in CRISP-ML(Q) requires the definition of requirements and constraints (e.g., performance, data quality requirements, model robustness, etc.), instantiation of the specific tasks (e.g., ML algorithm selection, model training, etc.), and specification of risks that might negatively impact the efficiency and success of the ML application (e.g., bias, overfitting, lack of reproducibility, etc.), quality assurance methods to mitigate risks when these risks need to be diminished.

3.1 Constraints and success criteria

3.1.1 Constraints

Over the past few years, there has been a challenge in the biological variables when it comes to mental illness. According to Lawrie et al. [16], practical issues such as the optimal combination of clinical and biological variables are being addressed, but the application of predictive algorithms to individuals or in routine clinical settings has yet to be tested. The development of predictive methods in mental health comes with substantial ethical questions, including whether people wish to know their level of risk, as well as individual and societal attitudes to the potential adverse effects of data sharing, early diagnosis, and treatment, which so far have been largely ignored [16].

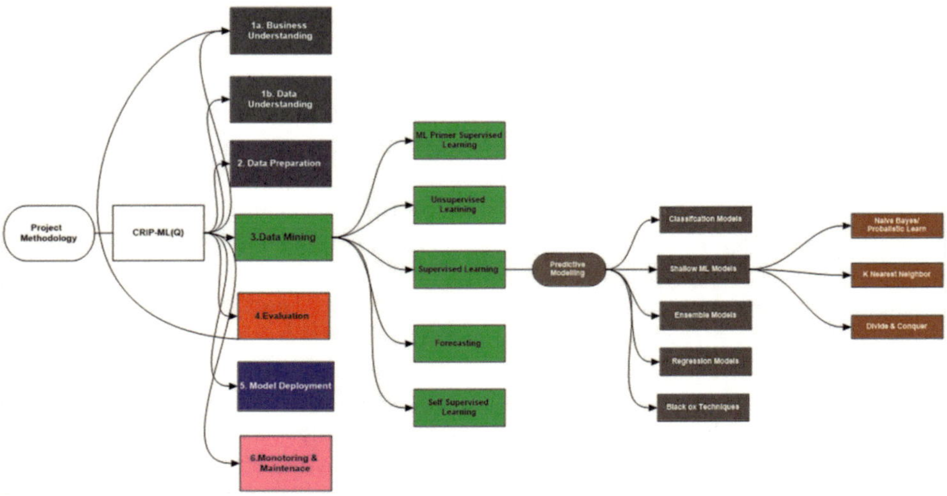

Figure 2.
CRISP-ML(Q) lifecycle.

3.1.2 Success criteria

The CRISP-ML is a model that has a guarantee of a 97% success rate in any given machine learning project, according to Studer et al. [17]; the other 3% is reserved for the failure rate. This is sort of a motivation to us because it gives a level of comfort when it comes to the feasibility of the study. Throughout the phases of the project development, the success criteria will be monitored, and whenever a risk is identified, adequate quality assurance measures are going to be implemented, which involves QA adoption from IEEE 730–1998. This innovative concept will help to decrease suicide rates, thus reducing resources channeled toward trauma counseling. The funds used by relatives to treat anxiety and depression will be redirected to help the family develop itself. It will also eliminate the expense of burying a loved one because of the reduction in suicide rates.

4. Analysis and model design

4.1 Introduction

The structure of the study followed the CRISP-ML(Q). This method has six (6) phases, and in this session, we are going to outline what was covered in each of the phases. The dataset was obtained from the Ministry of Health in Eswatini through HMIS.

4.1.1 Business and data understanding

4.1.1.1 Business understanding

Mental illness is significant and rising not only in the country but also in the whole world. In Eswatini, mental illness is a threat, and the need for mental health services is extremely high. Small-scale studies attest to the fact that common mental disorders such as depression, anxiety, and substance use are highly prevalent in the population of Eswatini. The treatment gap for mental disorders is large in the country. According to the "National Mental Health Strategy and Implementing Plan 2020–2025," there are no or limited nurse-led mental health services provided at regional hospitals, health centers, and clinics, yet the need is very high. From a few studies, it has been discovered that untreated common mental disorders (CMD) are the leading risk factor for suicide and attempted suicide. Based on the above-mentioned understanding, an innovative, proactive concept is of paramount importance in mitigating mental illnesses in the Kingdom of Eswatini.

4.1.1.2 Data understanding

Exploratory data analysis (EDA) is used by data scientists to analyze and investigate data sets and summarize their main characteristics, often employing data visualization methods. It helps determine how best to manipulate data sources to get the answers you need, making it easier for data scientists to discover patterns, spot anomalies, test a hypothesis, or check assumptions. The main purpose of EDA is to help look at data before making any assumptions. It can help identify obvious errors, as well as better understand patterns within the data, detect outliers or anomalous events, and find interesting relations among the variables as presented in **Figure 3**.

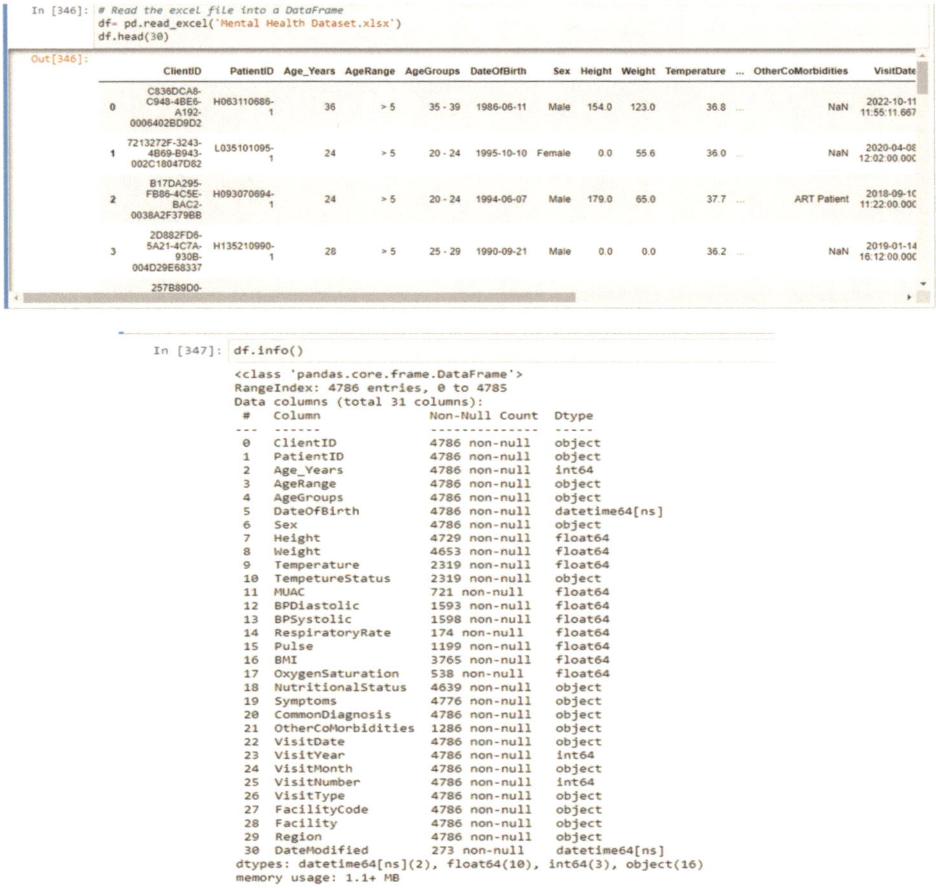

```
In [346]: # Read the excel file into a DataFrame
          df= pd.read_excel('Mental Health Dataset.xlsx')
          df.head(30)
Out[346]:
```

	ClientID	PatientID	Age_Years	AgeRange	AgeGroups	DateOfBirth	Sex	Height	Weight	Temperature	...	OtherCoMorbidities	VisitDate
0	C836DCA8-C948-4BE6-A192-0006402BD9D2	H063110686-1	36	> 5	35 - 39	1986-06-11	Male	154.0	123.0	36.8	...	NaN	2022-10-11 11:55:11.667
1	7213272F-3243-4B69-B943-002C18047D82	L035101095-1	24	> 5	20 - 24	1995-10-10	Female	0.0	55.6	36.0	...	NaN	2020-04-08 12:02:00.000
2	B17DA295-FB86-4C5E-BAC2-0038A2F379BB	H093070694-1	24	> 5	20 - 24	1994-06-07	Male	179.0	65.0	37.7	...	ART Patient	2018-09-10 11:22:00.000
3	2D882FD6-5A21-4C7A-930B-004D29E68337	H135210990-1	28	> 5	25 - 29	1990-09-21	Male	0.0	0.0	36.2	...	NaN	2019-01-14 16:12:00.000
	257B89D0-												

```
In [347]: df.info()
<class 'pandas.core.frame.DataFrame'>
RangeIndex: 4786 entries, 0 to 4785
Data columns (total 31 columns):
 #   Column               Non-Null Count  Dtype
---  ------               --------------  -----
 0   ClientID             4786 non-null   object
 1   PatientID            4786 non-null   object
 2   Age_Years            4786 non-null   int64
 3   AgeRange             4786 non-null   object
 4   AgeGroups            4786 non-null   object
 5   DateOfBirth          4786 non-null   datetime64[ns]
 6   Sex                  4786 non-null   object
 7   Height               4729 non-null   float64
 8   Weight               4653 non-null   float64
 9   Temperature          2319 non-null   float64
 10  TempetureStatus      2319 non-null   object
 11  MUAC                 721 non-null    float64
 12  BPDiastolic          1593 non-null   float64
 13  BPSystolic           1598 non-null   float64
 14  RespiratoryRate      174 non-null    float64
 15  Pulse                1199 non-null   float64
 16  BMI                  3765 non-null   float64
 17  OxygenSaturation     538 non-null    float64
 18  NutritionalStatus    4639 non-null   object
 19  Symptoms             4776 non-null   object
 20  CommonDiagnosis      4786 non-null   object
 21  OtherCoMorbidities   1286 non-null   object
 22  VisitDate            4786 non-null   object
 23  VisitYear            4786 non-null   int64
 24  VisitMonth           4786 non-null   object
 25  VisitNumber          4786 non-null   int64
 26  VisitType            4786 non-null   object
 27  FacilityCode         4786 non-null   object
 28  Facility             4786 non-null   object
 29  Region               4786 non-null   object
 30  DateModified         273 non-null    datetime64[ns]
dtypes: datetime64[ns](2), float64(10), int64(3), object(16)
memory usage: 1.1+ MB
```

Figure 3.
General information about the dataset.

```
In [355]: # The shape of the dataset
          df.shape

Out[355]: (4786, 31)
```

Figure 4.
The shape of the dataset.

The given dataset for this study has been extracted from the CMIS through the Ministry of Health in Eswatini. It has 31 columns, as shown in **Figure 4**.

Figure 4 shows the shape of the entire given dataset, which is (4786, 31).

Figure 5 shows that the dataset has some null values that need to be dealt with in the data pre-processing stage.

In terms of duplicates, the dataset looked good at a glance in **Figure 6**, but the deep investigation had to be done during the data pre-processing stage.

```
In [348]: df.isna().sum()

Out[348]: ClientID                0
          PatientID               0
          Age_Years               0
          AgeRange                0
          AgeGroups               0
          DateOfBirth             0
          Sex                     0
          Height                 57
          Weight                133
          Temperature          2467
          TempetureStatus      2467
          MUAC                 4065
          BPDiastolic          3193
          BPSystolic           3188
          RespiratoryRate      4612
          Pulse                3587
          BMI                  1021
          OxygenSaturation     4248
          NutritionalStatus     147
          Symptoms               10
          CommonDiagnosis         0
          OtherCoMorbidities   3500
          VisitDate               0
          VisitYear               0
          VisitMonth              0
          VisitNumber             0
          VisitType               0
          FacilityCode            0
          Facility                0
          Region                  0
          DateModified         4513
          dtype: int64
```

Figure 5.
Checking for null values.

```
In [351]: df.duplicated()

Out[351]: 0       False
          1       False
          2       False
          3       False
          4       False
                  ...
          4781    False
          4782    False
          4783    False
          4784    False
          4785    False
          Length: 4786, dtype: bool
```

Figure 6.
Checking for duplicates.

```
In [353]: total = df.isnull().sum().sort_values(ascending=False)
          percent = (df.isnull().sum()/df.isnull().count()).sort_values(ascending=False)
          missing_data = pd.concat([total, percent], axis=1, keys=['Total', 'Percent'])
          missing_data.head(20)
          print(missing_data)

                       Total   Percent
RespiratoryRate         4612  0.963644
DateModified            4513  0.942959
OxygenSaturation        4248  0.887589
MUAC                    4065  0.849352
Pulse                   3587  0.749478
OtherCoMorbidities      3500  0.731300
BPDiastolic             3193  0.667154
BPSystolic              3188  0.666109
Temperature             2467  0.515462
TempetureStatus         2467  0.515462
BMI                     1021  0.213331
NutritionalStatus        147  0.030715
Weight                   133  0.027789
Height                    57  0.011910
Symptoms                  10  0.002089
Region                     0  0.000000
VisitYear                  0  0.000000
Facility                   0  0.000000
FacilityCode               0  0.000000
VisitType                  0  0.000000
VisitNumber                0  0.000000
VisitMonth                 0  0.000000
DateOfBirth                0  0.000000
VisitDate                  0  0.000000
CommonDiagnosis            0  0.000000
Sex                        0  0.000000
Age_Years                  0  0.000000
PatientID                  0  0.000000
AgeRange                   0  0.000000
AgeGroups                  0  0.000000
ClientID                   0  0.000000
```

Figure 7.
Displaying variables with null values.

```
In [364]: sns.countplot(x ='Sex', data = df)
Out[364]: <Axes: xlabel='Sex', ylabel='count'>
```

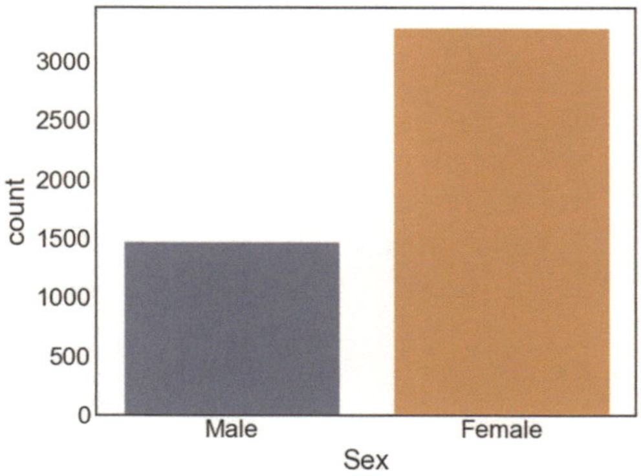

Figure 8.
Classification of mental illnesses based on gender.

Figure 7 shows the variables with null values in ascending order, starting with the highest.

Figure 8 shows the classification of mental illnesses based on gender.

Figure 9 shows the impact of mental illnesses across the four regions (Hhohho, Manzini, Lubombo, and Shiselweni) of Eswatini, with Manzini as the leading region and Lubombo with the least number of cases. The main reason why the only psychiatric center is located in Manzini.

Figure 10 shows the distribution and density by age of mental illnesses. The 120 years appeared to be an outlier, which is something that had to be dealt with during the data pre-processing stage.

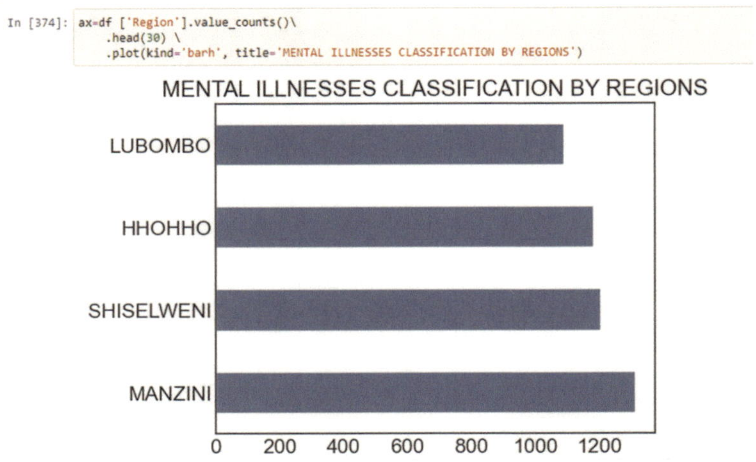

Figure 9.
Classification of mental illnesses by region.

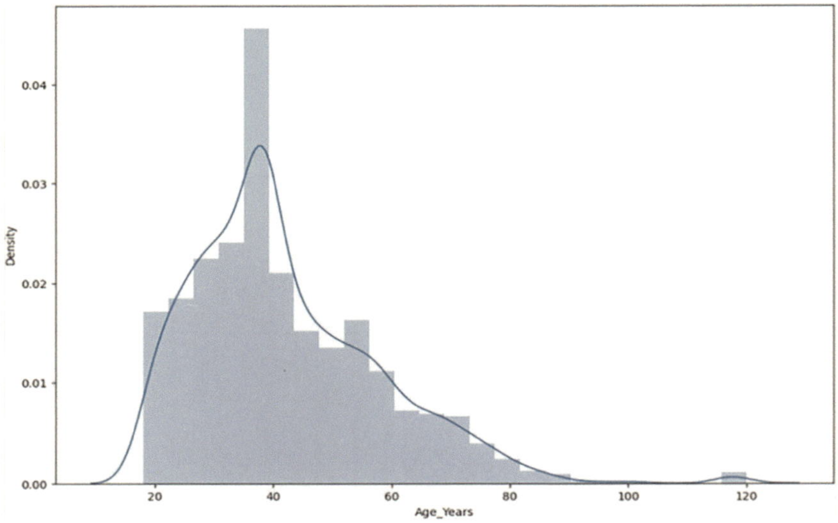

Figure 10.
Distribution and density by age with outliers.

Figure 11 shows the dominant mental illnesses in Eswatini. It can be seen that anxiety is the most dominant mental illness, followed by depression, and then schizophrenia and bipolar disorder.

4.1.2 Data preparation

This is a step that involved the transformation of raw data so that issues owing to the incompleteness or missing data, inconsistency, and lack of appropriate representation of trends were resolved in order to achieve a dataset that was in an understandable format.

```
ax= df ['CommonDiagnosis'].value_counts()\
    .head() \
    .plot(kind='barh', title='DOMINENT MENTAL ILLNESES (ESWATINI)')
```

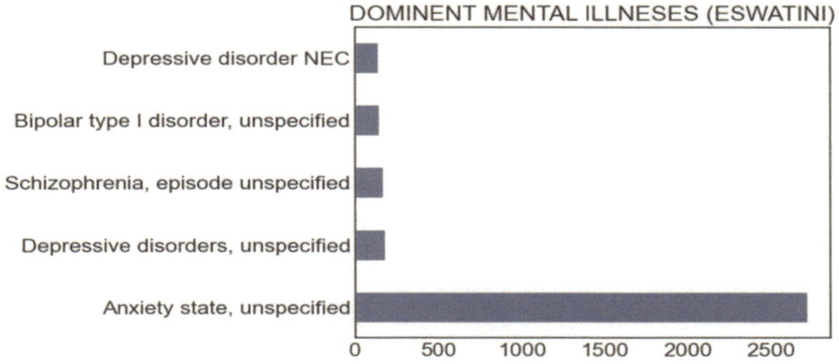

Figure 11.
Dominant mental illnesses in Eswatini.

4.1.2.1 Data redundancy

a. *Irrelevant attributes:* Some attributes in the dataset, such as "ClientID," are not important when performing data mining tasks; thus, they were dropped from the dataset, as shown in **Figure 12**.

b. *Duplicate data attributes:* Duplicates are usually present in the information contained in one or more other attributes. Apart from detecting redundancies between attributes, duplication was also detected at the tuple level. The duplicates were corrected or eliminated where necessary, as shown in **Figure 13**.

4.1.3 Data cleaning

This process was applied to the data by filling in missing values, smoothing the noisy data, resolving the inconsistency, and removing outliers.

```
In [382]: #Let's get rid of the variable "ClientID" .(Data reduction)
          data = df.drop(['ClientID'], axis= 1)

          data.isnull().sum().max() #just checking that there's no missing data missing...
          data.head(5)
```

Figure 12.
Dropping certain attributes.

```
In [461]: data.duplicated()

Out[461]: 0       False
          1       False
          2       False
          3       False
          4       False
                  ...
          4781    False
          4782    False
          4783    False
          4784    False
          4785    False
          Length: 4786, dtype: bool
```

Figure 13.
Detecting duplicate attributes.

a. *Missing values:* In this study, all null values were viewed in ascending order to have a clear view.

After identifying the missing values as shown in **Figure 14**, the attribute mean and attribute median were employed to fill in the missing values as shown in **Figure 15**.

b. *Removing or dealing with the outliers for the Age_year attribute:* The 120-year age was found to be an outlier, as shown in **Figure 16**, and was dropped from the dataset to smoothen the data in **Figure 17**.

c. *Dealing with not a number (NaN) values:* NaN (not a number) values were dealt with as some were replaced by zero, and others were replaced with the mean or median, as shown in **Figure 18**.

4.1.4 Visualization

For a better understanding and appreciation of all the techniques and algorithms we have employed during the data pre-processing stage, we employed the Walker Library for data visualization, as shown in **Figure 19**.

```
In [383]: #missing data
          total = data.isnull().sum().sort_values(ascending=False)
          percent = (data.isnull().sum()/data.isnull().count()).sort_values(ascending=Fal:
          missing_data = pd.concat([total, percent], axis=1, keys=['Total', 'Percent'])
          missing_data.head(20)
          print(missing_data)

                               Total   Percent
          RespiratoryRate       4612  0.963644
          DateModified          4513  0.942959
          OxygenSaturation      4248  0.887589
          MUAC                  4065  0.849352
          Pulse                 3587  0.749478
          OtherCoMorbidities    3500  0.731300
          BPDiastolic           3193  0.667154
          BPSystolic            3188  0.666109
          Temperature           2467  0.515462
          TempetureStatus       2467  0.515462
          BMI                   1021  0.213331
          NutritionalStatus      147  0.030715
          Weight                 133  0.027789
          Height                  57  0.011910
          Symptoms                10  0.002089
          VisitYear                0  0.000000
          Region                   0  0.000000
          Facility                 0  0.000000
          FacilityCode             0  0.000000
          VisitType                0  0.000000
          VisitNumber              0  0.000000
          VisitMonth               0  0.000000
          AgeRange                 0  0.000000
          VisitDate                0  0.000000
          CommonDiagnosis          0  0.000000
          AgeGroups                0  0.000000
          Age_Years                0  0.000000
          DateOfBirth              0  0.000000
          Sex                      0  0.000000
          PatientID                0  0.000000
```

Figure 14.
Viewing missing values.

```
In [459]: #complete missing age with mean
          data['Age_Years'].fillna(data['Age_Years'].median(), inplace = True)

          # Fill with media() values < 18 and > 120
          s = pd.Series(data['Age_Years'])
          s[s<18] = data['Age_Years'].median()
          data['Age_Years'] = s
          s = pd.Series(data['Age_Years'])
          s[s>120] = data['Age_Years'].median()
          data['Age_Years'] = s

          #Ranges of Age
          data['AgeRange'] = pd.cut(data['Age_Years'], [0,20,30,65,100], labels=["0-20", "21-30", "31-65", "66-100"], include_lowest=True)

In [460]: data.isna().sum()

          BPSystolic                 0
          RespiratoryRate            0
          Pulse                      0
          Body Mass Index            0
          OxygenSaturation           0
          NutritionalStatus          0
          Symptoms                   0
          CommonDiagnosis            0
          OtherCoMorbidities         0
          VisitDate                  0
          VisitYear                  0
          VisitMonth                 0
          VisitNumber                0
          VisitType                  0
          FacilityCode               0
          Facility                   0
          Region                     0
          DateModified            4513
          dtype: int64
```

Figure 15.
Filling in the missing values.

```
In [466]: ## Cleaning the age column remove outliers
          med_age = data[(data['Age_Years'] >= 18) | (data['Age_Years'] <= 75)]['Age_Years'].median()
          data['Age_Years'].replace(to_replace = data[(data['Age_Years'] < 18) | (data['Age_Years'] > 75)]['Age_Years'].tolist(),
                                    value = med_age, inplace = True)
```

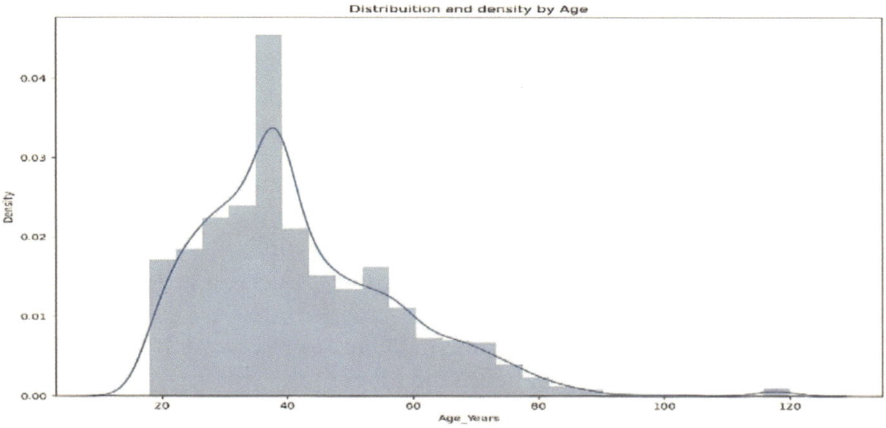

Figure 16.
Checking for outliers.

4.2 Data mining

4.2.1 Interesting patterns

Manzini is the leading region in the Kingdom of Eswatini, as shown in **Figure 20**, with people affected by mental health illnesses while the Lubombo region is the least affected.

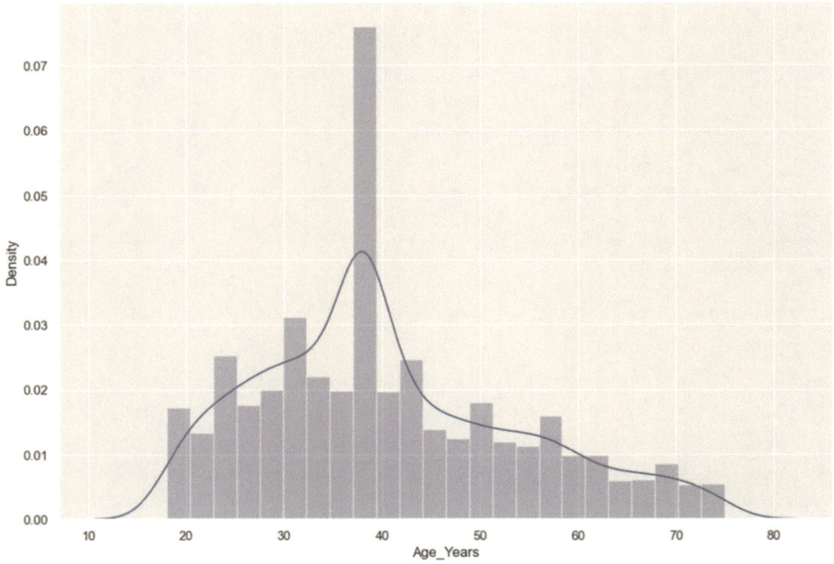

Figure 17.
Distribution and density by age without outliers.

```
[411]: #Replace "NaN" string from defaultString (Temperature column)
       data['Temperature'] = data['Temperature'].replace([defaultString], '0')
       print(data['Temperature'].unique())

       [36.8 36.0 37.7 36.2 36.5 '0' 36.9 36.3 38.3 35.8 37.0 36.1 35.7 36.7 36.4
        35.2 34.4 35.0 35.9 34.0 34.8 33.7 37.8 37.2 37.1 36.6 367.0 35.6 35.1
        35.4 35.5 37.3 33.3 32.6 37.6 33.2 34.7 39.0 34.6 35.3 37.4 37.5 32.7
        34.3 34.2 32.4 30.3 37.9 33.8 40.0 62.2 34.1 33.9 32.0 33.0 39.8 327.0
        38.0 39.7 34.5 355.0 34.9 33.1 32.9 39.3 32.5 33.4 331.0 39.1 38.4 32.1
        38.5 38.8 31.2 33.6 32.2 38.2 360.4 371.0]
```

Figure 18.
Dealing with empty attributes.

Figure 21 visualizes the distribution of mental illnesses against the different age groups in the Kingdom of Eswatini. It is worth noting that the 40-year-old age group is the most affected group in the Kingdom of Eswatini, which is a great concern since this is the most economically active group. On average, the most affected age groups range from 17 years to 60 years.

Figure 22 shows the classification of mental illnesses in Eswatini. The leading illnesses are anxiety and depression, hence the focus of the study.

Figure 23 shows the classification of mental illnesses based on gender. From **Figure 23**, it is worth noting that females are the most affected by mental illnesses.

4.3 Data splitting

Most of the target variables, as shown in **Figure 24**, were object data types. The object data type cannot be used in its present state for modeling; in order to tackle this issue, transformation must take place. We had to transform them through label encoding.

We converted the first two mental illnesses from strings to integers by assigning 0 to anxiety and 1 to depression, as shown in **Figure 25**.

Through LabelEncoder, as shown in **Figure 26**, the other x-values were transformed from either strings or floats into integers.

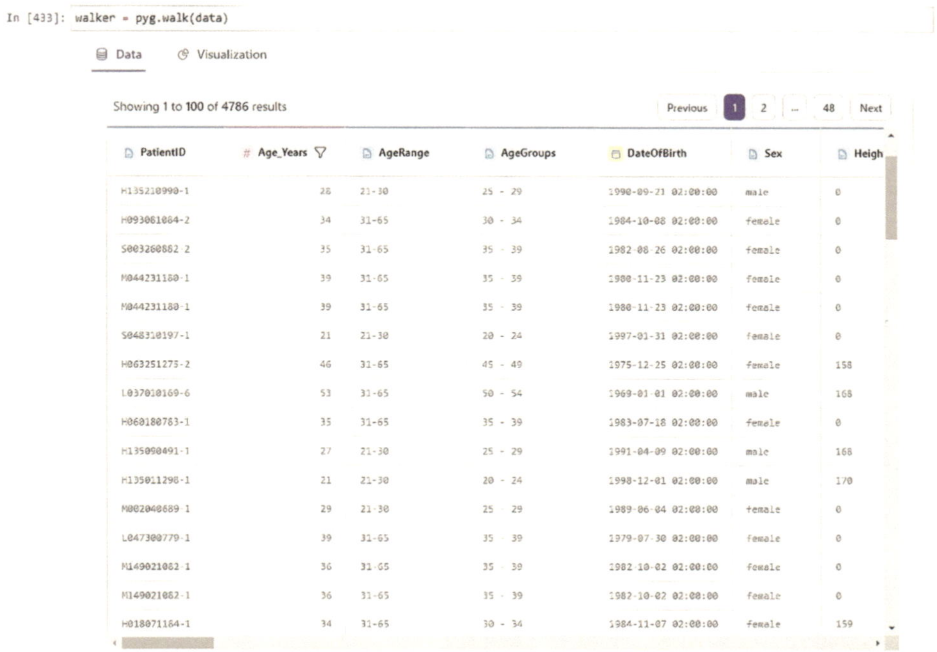

```
In [433]: walker = pyg.walk(data)
```

Data   Visualization

Showing 1 to 100 of 4786 results   Previous 1 2 ... 48 Next

PatientID	Age_Years	AgeRange	AgeGroups	DateOfBirth	Sex	Heigh
H135210990-1	28	21-30	25 - 29	1990-09-21 02:00:00	male	0
H093061084-2	34	31-65	30 - 34	1984-10-08 02:00:00	female	0
S003260882-2	35	31-65	35 - 39	1982-08-26 02:00:00	female	0
M044231180-1	39	31-65	35 - 39	1980-11-23 02:00:00	female	0
M044231180-1	39	31-65	35 - 39	1980-11-23 02:00:00	female	0
S048310197-1	21	21-30	20 - 24	1997-01-31 02:00:00	female	0
H063251275-2	46	31-65	45 - 49	1975-12-25 02:00:00	female	158
L037010169-6	53	31-65	50 - 54	1969-01-01 02:00:00	male	168
H060180783-1	35	31-65	35 - 39	1983-07-18 02:00:00	female	0
H135090491-1	27	21-30	25 - 29	1991-04-09 02:00:00	male	168
H135011298-1	21	21-30	20 - 24	1998-12-01 02:00:00	male	170
M002040689-1	29	21-30	25 - 29	1989-06-04 02:00:00	female	0
L047300779-1	39	31-65	35 - 39	1979-07-30 02:00:00	female	0
M149021082-1	36	31-65	35 - 39	1982-10-02 02:00:00	female	0
M149021082-1	36	31-65	35 - 39	1982-10-02 02:00:00	female	0
H018071164-1	34	31-65	30 - 34	1984-11-07 02:00:00	female	159

Figure 19.
The Walker Library for data visualization.

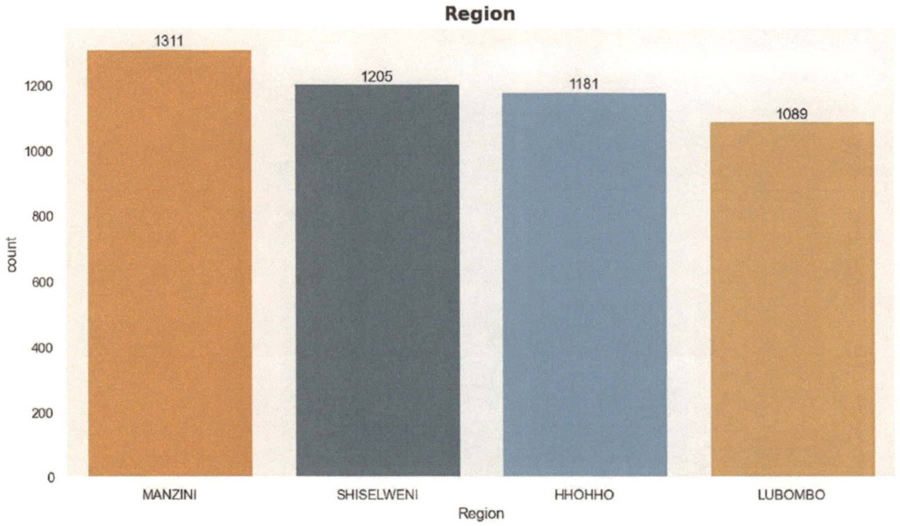


```
In [281]: #Total Mental illness cases as per region
          data['Region'].value_counts()

Out[281]: MANZINI       1311
          SHISELWENI    1205
          HHOHHO        1181
          LUBOMBO       1089
          Name: Region, dtype: int64
```

Figure 20.
The distribution of mental health illnesses across the country.

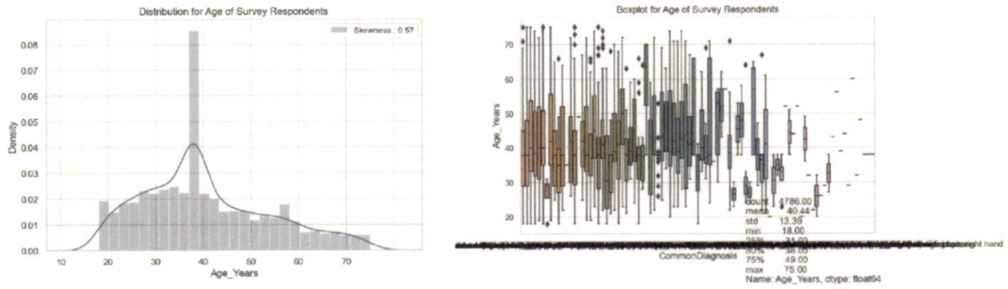

(a) (b)

Figure 21.
Distribution and boxplot for age of survey respondents.

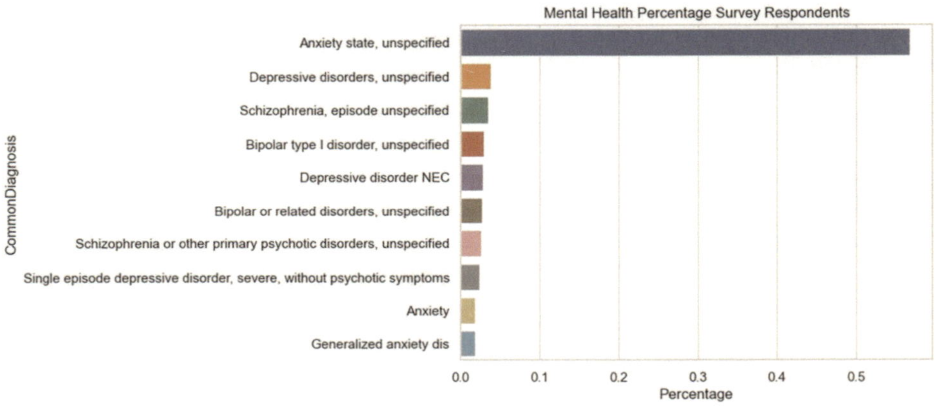

Figure 22.
Mental health survey respondents.

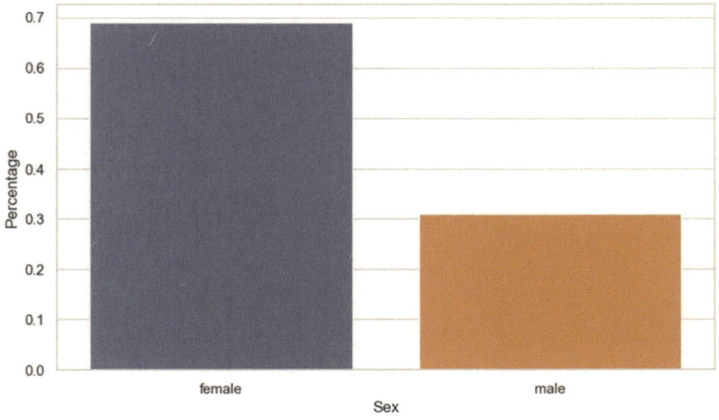

Figure 23.
Survey respondents by gender.

```
 0   ClientID            3183 non-null   object
 1   PatientID           3183 non-null   object
 2   Age_Years           3183 non-null   int64
 3   AgeRange            3183 non-null   object
 4   AgeGroups           3183 non-null   object
 5   DateOfBirth         3183 non-null   datetime64[ns]
 6   Sex                 3183 non-null   object
 7   Height              3162 non-null   float64
 8   Weight              3117 non-null   float64
 9   Temperature         1405 non-null   float64
 10  TempetureStatus     1405 non-null   object
 11  MUAC                576 non-null    float64
 12  BMI                 3183 non-null   float64
 13  BPDiastolic         586 non-null    float64
 14  Symptoms            3183 non-null   int64
 15  CommonDiagnosis     3183 non-null   int64
 16  OtherCoMorbidities  848 non-null    object
 17  VisitDate           3183 non-null   object
 18  VisitYear           3183 non-null   int64
 19  VisitMonth          3183 non-null   object
 20  VisitNumber         3183 non-null   int64
 21  VisitType           3183 non-null   object
 22  FacilityCode        3183 non-null   object
 23  Facility            3183 non-null   object
 24  Region              3183 non-null   object
 25  DateModified        229 non-null    datetime64[ns]
dtypes: datetime64[ns](2), float64(6), int64(5), object(13)
memory usage: 646.7+ KB
```

Figure 24.
Label encoding.

```
In [67]:  1 df['CommonDiagnosis'].replace({'Anxiety state, unspecified':0,'Depressive disorders, unspecified':1}, inplace=True)

In [68]:  1 df['CommonDiagnosis'].unique()
Out[68]: array([0, 1], dtype=int64)
```

Figure 25.
Transforming common diagnoses for mental illness classification.

We then split the dataset into training and testing with a ratio of 20%:80%. Our X-values entail ('Age_Years', 'Encoded_Gender', 'Encoded_Height', 'Encoded_Weight', 'Encoded_Temperaure', 'Encoded_BMI', 'Symptoms').

For the dependent variable, we selected 'CommonDiagnosis' for training the model, as shown in **Figure 27**.

4.3.1 Model evaluation

In this study, four algorithms were compared, including Logistic Regression, Decision Tree Classifier, Random Forest Classifier and AdaBoost Classifier. From the results in **Figure 28**, the Random Forest classifier outperforms the other three in terms of accuracy, with 96% accuracy.

```
In [237]:


# Encoding the 'Gender' categorical variable
le = LabelEncoder()
df['Encoded_Gender'] = le.fit_transform(df['Sex'])

# Encoding the 'Height' categorical variable

df['Encoded_Height'] = le.fit_transform(df['Height'])

# Encoding the 'Weight' categorical variable

df['Encoded_Weight'] = le.fit_transform(df['Weight'])


# Encoding the 'Temperature' categorical variable

df['Encoded_Temperature'] = le.fit_transform(df['Temperature'])


# Encoding the 'TempetureStatus' categorical variable

df['Encoded_BMI'] = le.fit_transform(df['BMI'])

```

Figure 26.
Label encoding of x-values.

```
]:
# Importing necessary Libraries
from sklearn.model_selection import train_test_split
from sklearn.metrics import mean_squared_error, r2_score
# Selecting the random features and target
X = df[['Age_Years', 'Encoded_Gender', 'Encoded_Height','Encoded_Weight','Encoded_Temperature','Encoded_BMI','Symptoms']]
#'Encoded_MUAC','Encoded_Pulse']]
y = df['CommonDiagnosis']
```

```
]:
# Splitting the Dataset
X_train, X_test, y_train, y_test = train_test_split(X, y, test_size=0.2,random_state=42)
```

```
]:
X_train_filled = X_train.fillna(0)
# Fill missing values with zero in the testing set
X_test_filled = X_test.fillna(0)
```

Figure 27.
Data splitting.

4.3.2 Confusion matrix

The confusion matrix provides a comprehensive overview of model performance: It goes beyond simple accuracy measures by displaying how often the model correctly and incorrectly classifies instances for each class. This allows for a nuanced understanding of the model's behavior across different categories.

Figure 29 shows that 84% of the anxiety predictions were accurate, while only 12% of the depression predictions were accurate. The huge difference between the two predictions is due to the features that were selected before the feature selection algorithm was employed. We also discovered that 1% of the mental illnesses were predicted as depression, yet they were anxiety, and 3% were predicted as anxiety, yet they were depression. These false predictions had a huge impact on the low performance of the prediction score for depression because 3% of these predictions were classified as anxiety, yet they were depression.

```
In [227]:
model_dict = {}

model_dict['Logistic regression']= LogisticRegression (solver='liblinear', random_state=49)
model_dict[ 'Decision Tree Classifier' ] = DecisionTreeClassifier (random_state=49)
model_dict ['Random Forest Classifier'] = RandomForestClassifier (random_state=49)
model_dict ['AdaBoost Classifier' ] = AdaBoostClassifier (random_state=49)
```

```
In [223]:
def model_test (X_train, X_test, y_train, y_test, model, model_name):
    model.fit(X_train,y_train)
    y_pred = model.predict (X_test)
    accuracy = accuracy_score (y_test,y_pred)
model_dict[ 'Decision Tree Classifier' ] = DecisionTreeClassifier (random_state=49)
model_dict ['Random Forest Classifier'] = RandomForestClassifier (random_state=49)
model_dict ['AdaBoost Classifier' ] = AdaBoostClassifier (random_state=49)
def model_test (X_train, X_test, y_train, y_test, model, model_name):
    model.fit(X_train,y_train)
    y_pred = model.predict (X_test)
    accuracy = accuracy_score (y_test,y_pred)
    print('===================================={}====================================='.format(model_name))
    print('Score is : {}'.format (accuracy))
    print()
for model_name, model in model_dict.items ():
    model_test(X_train, X_test, y_train, y_test, model,model_name)
    print('===================================={}====================================='.format(model_name))
    print()
    print()
```

```
====================================Logistic regression=====================================
Score is : 0.8555729984301413

====================================Logistic regression=====================================


====================================Decision Tree Classifier=====================================
Score is : 0.9466248037676609

====================================Decision Tree Classifier=====================================


====================================Random Forest Classifier=====================================
Score is : 0.9623233908948194

====================================Random Forest Classifier=====================================


====================================AdaBoost Classifier=====================================
Score is : 0.9529042386185244

====================================AdaBoost Classifier=====================================
```

Figure 28.
Random forest training results.

```
In [78]:
cf_matrix = confusion_matrix(y_test, y_pred)
sns.heatmap(cf_matrix/np.sum(cf_matrix), annot=True, fmt=' .2%')
plt.title( 'Confusion Matrix')
plt.xlabel('Predicted')
plt.ylabel('Actual')

Out[78]: Text(50.722222222222214, 0.5, 'Actual')
```

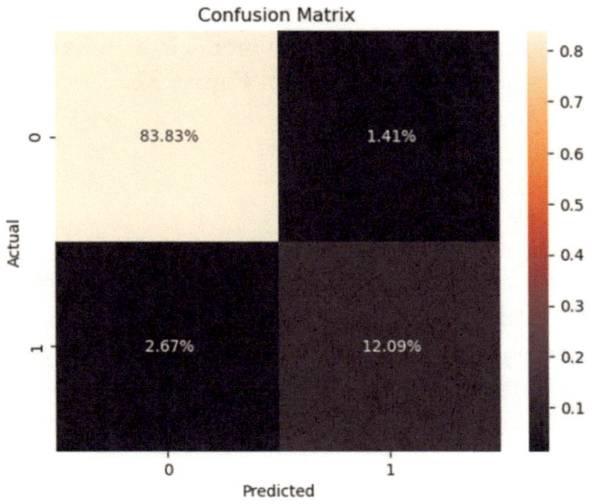

Figure 29.
Confusion matrix.

```
#CaLcuLate  the variance
X_train_v1.var(axis=0)
```

```
Age_Years                345.482370
Encoded_Gender             0.199604
Encoded_Height          1456.541232
Encoded_Weight         35536.924058
Encoded_Temperature      299.796871
Encoded_BMI           110063.902697
Symptoms                 101.510639
dtype: float64
```

Figure 30.
Selecting important features.

4.3.3 Feature selection

The goal of feature selection is to select a subset of j features that a classifier uses to reach optimal performance, where j is a user-defined parameter. We used a threshold variance to select important features after evaluating the performance of the model.

Figure 30 shows that indeed there is a huge variance between the variables. To counteract this problem, we employed a MinMaxScaler library to smooth the variance.

From **Figure 31**, it is worth noting that for detecting depression and anxiety, important features include gender, height, weight, temperature, BMI, and symptoms.

4.3.4 Re-training the model with the most important features

After important feature selection based on the scores, the accuracy remains at 96%, which means eliminating age from the model has not had much impact on the accuracy or model performance, as shown in **Figure 32**.

4.4 Model building

4.4.1 Detecting depression

Depression disorder results from a combined effect of various physiological, environmental, psychological, and socioeconomic factors. Recent studies show that biological predictors of blood pressure levels, heart rate, and body mass index (BMI) are associated with depressive symptoms [18].

4.4.2 Detecting anxiety

Anxiety disorders are a common problem in adolescent mental health. According to Ref. [19], recent studies show that risk factors associated with general anxiety disorder include age, sex, temperature, BMI, and familial factors.

```python
from sklearn.preprocessing import MinMaxScaler
scaler = MinMaxScaler()
scaled_X_train_v1 = scaler.fit_transform(X_train_v1)
```

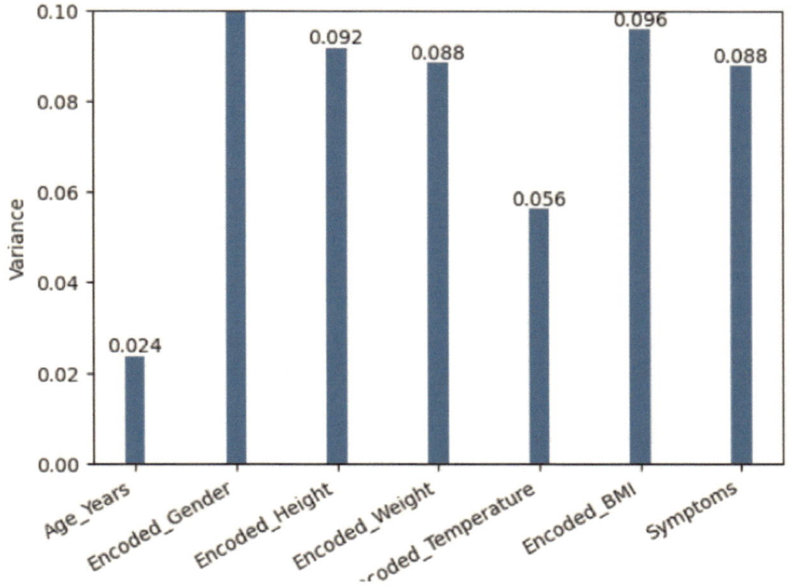

Figure 31.
MinMaxScaler.

```
=====================================Logistic regression======================================
Score is : 0.8555729984301413

=====================================Logistic regression======================================


=====================================Decision Tree Classifier=====================================
Score is : 0.9466248037676609

=====================================Decision Tree Classifier=====================================


=====================================Random Forest Classifier=====================================
Score is : 0.9623233908948194

=====================================Random Forest Classifier=====================================


=====================================AdaBoost Classifier======================================
Score is : 0.9529042386185244

=====================================AdaBoost Classifier======================================
```

Figure 32.
Performance of the algorithms after re-training.

From the above evaluations, it is worth mentioning that anxiety and depression in Eswatini can be predicted using Random Forest, which has an accuracy of 96%. The most important features of this model include gender, height, BMI, weight, and symptoms.

4.5 Model deployment

4.5.1 Model code

From the model evaluation, we selected the Random Forest algorithm based on its accuracy in developing the model. Because of the data set, all the models had a high false positive rate; hence, we opted to select the best model based on accuracy alone. Below is the code that has been used to deploy the trained model in the user interface using the Streamlit library and pickle.

```
# Importing libraries
import numpy as np
import streamlit as st
import pickle
# Loading the trained Model
loaded_model=pickle.load(open('C:/Users/Peso/Desktop/MENTAL/glo/FinalModel/model_pickle', 'rb'))
#creating a function model
def mentalhealth_preidiction(input_data):
  # changing the input data to nmpy array
  input_data_as_numpy_array = np.asarray(input_data)
  # changing the input data to nmpy array
  input_data_as_numpy_array = np.asarray(input_data)
  #reshape the array as we are predicting for one instance
  input_data_reshaped = input_data_as_numpy_array.reshape(1,-1)
  #reshape the array as we are predicting for one instance
  prediction = loaded_model.predict(input_data_reshaped)
  print(prediction)
  if (prediction[0]==0):
      return 'The Client is Sufffering from Anxiety'
  else:
    return 'The Client is Suffereing from Depression'
def main()
  #code for prediction
  diagnosis = ''
  st.title('Mental Health Predictive Web App')
  Age_Years = st.text_input('Age')
  Encoded_Gender = st.text_input('Gender')
  Encoded_Height = st.text_input('Height')
  Encoded_Weight = st.text_input('Weight')
  Encoded_Temperatures = st.text_input('Temperature')
  Encoded_BMI = st.text_input('BMI')
  Symptoms = st.text_input('Symptoms')
  # creating a button fro condition
  if st.button('Test Results'):
    diagnosis= mentalhealth_preidiction([Age_Years,Encoded_Gender,Encoded_Height,
    Encoded_Weight,Encoded_Temperatures,Encoded_BMI,Symptoms])
  st.success(diagnosis)
if __name__== '__main__':
  main()
```

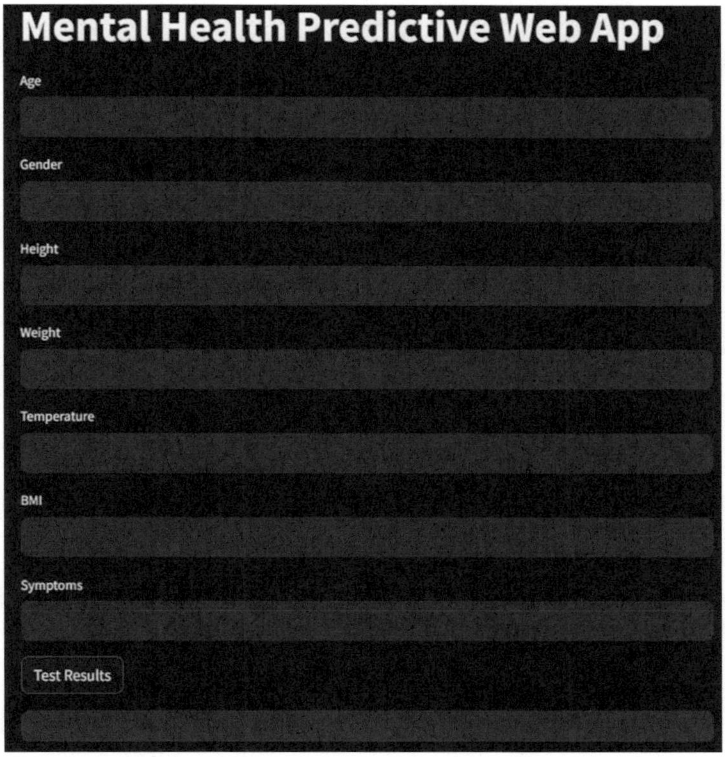

Figure 33.
The graphical user interface for monitoring and maintenance.

4.5.2 The graphical user Interface (GUI)

The web application uses Streamlit, and its model is run by the Random Forest algorithm for predicting anxiety and depression, as shown in **Figure 33**.

4.6 Monitoring and maintenance

In the ML lifecycle, even after the deployment stage. The model will undergo constant monitoring and maintenance in order to be able to evaluate the performance and accuracy of the model over time. This is because data is in a continual state of motion and keeps on changing, which might cause the model to degrade. In this study, the choice to automate the ML workflow to monitor and retrain the model constantly, which will ensure its longevity, is necessary.

4.6.1 Positive aspects

- *Early intervention*: Identifying individuals at risk of developing anxiety or depression can enable early intervention and prevent the progression of symptoms.

- *Personalization*: The ML model can analyze individual data, including factors like demographics, medical history, and social status, to tailor interventions and treatments.
- *Resource allocation*: Early prediction of mental illnesses across the different age groups can help the government and other stakeholders to allocate mental health resources more efficiently.
- *Accuracy*: This project has confirmed from the existing literature that indeed ML models can achieve high accuracy in predicting anxiety and depression.

4.6.2 Challenges to address

- *Poor data quality and biases*: ML models rely on good data, and biased data can lead to inaccurate predictions and exacerbate existing inequalities.
- *Privacy concerns*: Accessing and using sensitive mental health data raises ethical concerns and requires careful consideration of privacy and security.
- *Spectrum of the symptoms*: The symptoms of mental illnesses are not categorized or structured and are based on individual assumptions, which makes it very difficult to encode.
- *Validation of inputs in database systems*: The nature of the dataset shows that the systems used for inputting the data are not properly designed to enforce data validations.

5. Conclusion and recommendations

5.1 Conclusion

From this study, findings showed that early detection in identifying individuals at risk of developing anxiety or depression can enable early intervention and prevention. It is noted that ML models can analyze individual data, including factors like demographics and regions, just to mention a few, to tailor interventions and treatments. Such a technological intervention can help the government and other stakeholders in resource allocation. Finally, in terms of accuracy, Random Forest performed better than Logistic Regression, AdaBoost, and Decision Tree. This study has confirmed from the existing literature that indeed ML models can achieve a certain level of accuracy in predicting anxiety and depression.

Overall, while challenges remain, developing predictive ML models for anxiety and depression holds significant promise for improving mental health care. By addressing ethical concerns, prioritizing data quality and interpretability, and ensuring collaboration with healthcare professionals, we can leverage this technology to make a positive impact on the lives of EmaSwati.

5.2 Recommendations

- *Invest in education and training*: The MOH and other stakeholders need to equip healthcare professionals with skills to interpret and utilize ML tools effectively.

Additionally, an awareness program on the importance of data and information needs to be vigorously done across the different ministries and organizations in Eswatini in order for the country to move forward when it comes to data storage.

- *Develop transparent and interpretable models*: The government, through the MOH, has to prioritize explainable AI methods to enable trust and understanding of ML predictions in clinical settings and improve the Information and Communication Technology (ICT) infrastructure in clinics and hospitals across the country.

- *Collaborate with developers, clinicians, and mental health professionals*: There should be a close collaboration between developers, researchers, and healthcare practitioners for the practical and ethical implementation of innovation in the health sector.

- *Focus on ethical data collection and analysis*: Ensure diverse and unbiased datasets, implement anonymization procedures, and involve data subjects in research design.

Author details

Stephen Fashoto[1,2]*, Ndumiso Ginindza[1], Sibusiso Dlamini[1] and Olubunmi Fashoto[3]

1 Department of Computer Science, University of Eswatini, Kwaluseni, Eswatini

2 Department of Informatics, Namibia University of Science and Technology, Windhoek, Namibia

3 Department of Psychology, Eswatini Medical Christian University, Mbabane, Eswatini

*Address all correspondence to: gbengafash2@gmail.com

References

[1] Thieme A, Belgrave D, Doherty G. Machine learning in mental health: A systematic review of the HCI literature to support the development of effective and implementable ML systems. ACM Transactions on Computer-Human Interaction. 2020;**27**(5):1-53. Article Number 34. DOI: 10.1145/3398069

[2] Pengpid S, Peltzer K. The prevalence and correlates of suicidal ideation, plans and suicide attempts among 15-to 69-year-old persons in Eswatini. Behavioral Sciences. 2020;**10**(11):1-11. DOI: 10.3390/bs10110172

[3] Folorunso SO, Fashoto SG, Olaomi J, Fashoto OY. A multi-label learning model for psychotic diseases in Nigeria. Informatics in Medicine Unlocked. 2020; **19**:100326

[4] Rezaii N, Walker E, Wolff P. A machine learning approach to predicting psychosis using semantic density and latent content analysis. NPJ Schizophrenia. 2019;**5**(1):1-12

[5] Elujide OI, Fashoto SG, Fashoto OY, Mbunge E, Folorunso SO, Olamijuwon JO. Application of deep and machine learning techniques for multi-label classification performance on psychotic disorder diseases. In: Informatics in Medicine Unlocked. Vol. 23. United Kingdom: Elsevier; 2021. p. 100545

[6] Vieira S, Pinaya WHL, Mechelli A. Using deep learning to investigate the neuroimaging correlates of psychiatric and neurological disorders: Methods and applications. Neuroscience and Biobehavioral Reviews. 2017;**74**:58-75

[7] de Filippis R, Carbone EA, Gaetano R, Bruni A, Pugliese V, Segura-Garcia C, et al. Machine learning techniques in a structural and functional mri diagnostic approach in schizophrenia: A systematic review. Neuropsychiatric Disease and Treatment. 2019;**15**:1605

[8] Mental Health and Youth Unemployment – Separc. (n.d.). Available from: https://www.separc.co.sz/2019/06/11/mental-health-and-youth-unemployment/ [Accessed: July 2, 2023]

[9] Rahman RA, Omar K, Azman S, Noah M, Danuri M, Ali Al-Garadi M. Application of machine learning methods in mental health detection: A systematic review. IEEE Access. 2020;**8**: 183952-183964. DOI: 10.1109/ACCESS.2020.3029154

[10] Liu Y, Qu HQ, Mentch FD, Qu J, Chang X, Nguyen K, et al. Application of deep learning algorithm on whole genome sequencing data uncovers structural variants associated with multiple mental disorders in African American patients. Molecular Psychiatry. 2022;**27**(3):1469-1478. DOI: 10.1038/s41380-021-01418-1

[11] Su C, Xu Z, Pathak J, Wang F. Deep learning in mental health outcome research: A scoping review. Translational Psychiatry. 2020;**10**(1):1 -26. DOI: 10.1038/s41398-020-0780-3

[12] Freeman D, Reeve S, Robinson A, Ehlers A, Clark D, Spanlang B, et al. Virtual reality in the assessment, understanding, and treatment of mental health disorders. Psychological Medicine. 2017;**47**(14):2393-2400. DOI: 10.1017/S003329171700040X

[13] Garriga R, Mas J, Abraha S, Nolan J, Harrison O, Tadros G, et al. Machine learning model to predict mental health

crises from electronic health records. Nature Medicine. 2022;**28**(6):1240-1248. DOI: 10.1038/s41591-022-01811-5

[14] Madan S, Julius Zimmer F, Balabin H, Schaaf S, Fröhlich H, Fluck J, et al. Deep learning-based detection of psychiatric attributes from German mental health records. International Journal of Medical Informatics. 2022;**161** (November 2021):1-8. DOI: 10.1016/j.ijmedinf.2022.104724

[15] Sciences M, Ehsan D, Intelligent G. Mental health prediction models using machine learning in higher education. Turkish Journal of Computer And Mathematics Education. 2021;**12**(5): 1782-1792

[16] Lawrie SM, Fletcher-Watson S, Whalley HC, McIntosh AM. Predicting major mental illness: Ethical and practical considerations. BJPsych Open. 2019;**5**(2):1-5. DOI: 10.1192/BJO.2019.11

[17] Studer S, Bui TB, Drescher C, Hanuschkin A, Winkler L, Peters S, et al. Towards CRISP-ML (Q): A machine learning process model with quality assurance methodology. Machine Learning and Knowledge Extraction. 2021;**3**:392-413

[18] Hildrum B, Romild U, Holmen J. Anxiety and depression lowers blood pressure: 526 22-year follow-up of the population based HUNT study, Norway. BMC Public Health. 2011;**527**(11):601. DOI: 10.1186/1471-2458-11-601

[19] Narmandakh A, Roest AM, de Jonge P, Oldehinkel AJ. Psychosocial and biological risk factors of anxiety disorders in adolescents: A TRAILS report. European Child & Adolescent Psychiatry. 2021;**30**(12):1969-1982. DOI: 10.1007/s00787-020-01669-3. Epub 2020 Oct 28

Chapter 9

Exploring Risk Factors for Offending Behaviours in Individuals with Psychosis and Impact of Interventions to Reduce Offending

Armita Adily, Stephen Allnutt and Tony Butler

Abstract

A relatively high proportion of offenders suffer from mental illness, including conditions such as psychosis. The association between psychosis and offending behaviour was investigated in a population-based study in Australia. Findings from this work have implications for policy and practice in the management of people in the criminal justice arena to reduce reoffending in those diagnosed with psychosis. This chapter summarises the key findings from this body of work, including the association between psychosis and offending, risk factors for reoffending, and the impacts of court diversion and treatment by mental health services in reducing reoffending rates in people with psychosis. This chapter highlights the characteristics of vulnerable groups with psychosis who have reduced access to preventive interventions and are thus at higher risk of offending. The identified gaps in access to effective interventions for at-risk groups highlight the need to address equitable access for all.

Keywords: psychosis, offending, reoffending, court diversion, mental health services

1. Introduction

Psychosis is a mental disorder characterised by poor reality testing that can contribute to offending behaviour. Psychotic symptoms such as delusions and hallucinations, along with cognitive impairments that can coexist, distort reality perception and influence decision-making behind behaviours that may violate laws or social norms and attract the attention of the police.

Studies have consistently shown that psychosis is a risk factor for criminal offending, including violent offending [1–7]. Offenders with mental illness, including those diagnosed with psychosis, are known to be an increased risk of reoffending and returning to the criminal justice system than those without psychosis [4].

Sensationalist media focus on this issue has resulted in a perception that those with mental illness are likely to engage in violence and thus pose a risk to the community.

Reducing recidivism has been a challenge for the criminal justice system in Australia, as over half of prisoners (52%) return to prison within two years of release [8]. Interventions are needed to prevent this reoffending trajectory.

Studies show that the extent to which psychosis contributes to offending behaviour varies depending on factors, such as different treatment practices, legislation, and allocation of resources for mental health treatment and services in each jurisdiction [9, 10]. The high rate of reoffending in Australia has led to calls for the development of evidence-based programs to reduce offending [11], including reducing the incarceration rate of Australian Aboriginal people, which is believed to be the highest of any Indigenous group in the world. Part of this effort to reduce offending behaviour involved research to better understand the relationship between psychosis, treatment, and offending to better inform policy development.

The body of work described in this chapter involved several studies to examine the impact of existing practices to reduce reoffending by people with psychosis, including a court diversion program established in New South Wales (NSW) to divert those with serious mental illness into treatment rather than incarceration, and the impact of contact with community mental health services on offending within a 14-year follow-up. NSW is Australia's most populous state and houses 30% of prisoners in the country, of whom 30% are Aboriginal [12].

Researchers from the University of New South Wales, Sydney undertook a retrospective cohort study involving population-level linkage of eight administrative data collections in NSW, including: Admitted Patient Data Collection (APDC), Emergency Department Data Collection (EDDC), Mental Health Ambulatory Data Collection (MH-AMB), Pharmaceutical Drugs of Addiction System (PHDAS), Reoffending Database (RoD), Offender Integrated Management System (OIMS), Registry of Births, Deaths & Marriages (RBDM) deaths data, and Australian Bureau of Statistics (ABS) mortality data (**Figure 1**). The study population comprised two cohorts: (1) all individuals diagnosed with psychosis on admission to a hospital or presentation to an emergency department in NSW between 1 July 2001 and 30 December 2012, and (2) all individuals who had committed at least one offence between 1 July 2001 and 31 December 2015. The age- and sex-matched controls were selected from the NSW Ministry of Health data (see Section 2.1). Detailed information on the methods is described elsewhere [1, 13, 14]. In this chapter, we summarise some of the major findings from three of the publications based on the data linkage study [1, 13, 14].

First, we present findings on the socio-demographic and criminographic factors in the complex relationship between psychosis and offending. While the relationship between psychosis and offending is compelling, the mechanisms underlying this relationship are complex and not well explained by empirical studies. Moreover, much of the evidence has focused on the association between serious mental illness and violent offending and less attention has been given to the relationship with other offence types.

Serious mental illness is associated with an increased likelihood of having criminogenic factors, which are also found in non-mentally ill offender populations, such as homelessness, poor social and personal relationships, unemployment, substance use, poor education attainment, and antisocial behaviours [1]. It has been suggested that, in many instances, mental health symptomology does not have direct causal effect on most offending behaviour [15]. Although symptoms of mental illness have not been found to be strong predictors for offending behaviours, modest associations were found [16]. Bonta et al. ([16], p. 278) state that *"from both a risk prediction and a recidivism reduction perspective, symptoms of mental illness do not appear*

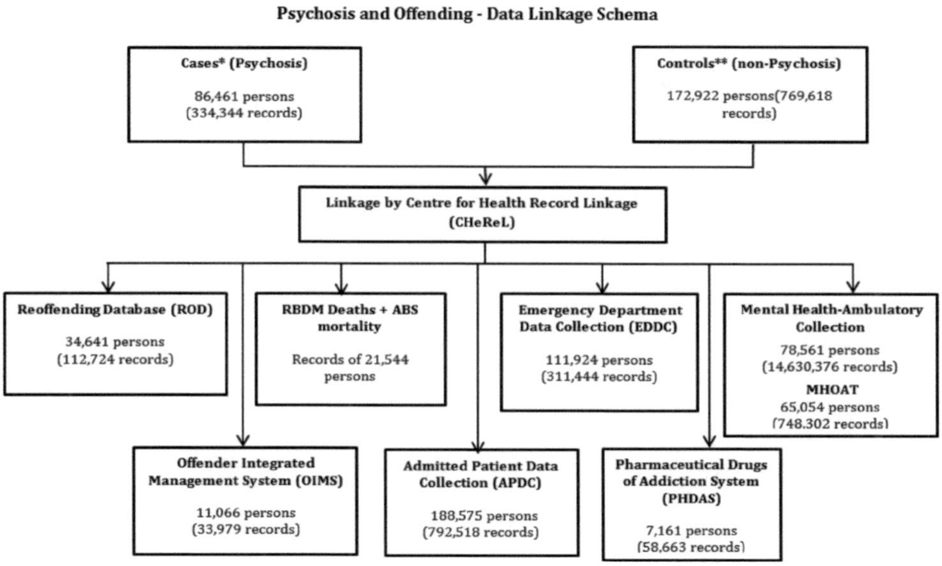

Figure 1.
*The linked data to examine the association between psychosis and offending in NSW. Linkage by the NSW Centre for Health Record Linkage (CheReL). *Psychosis cases selected from the APDC and EDDC data collections—2001–2012 (EDDC—2005 onwards). **Controls selected from CHeReL's master linkage key (2 controls for each psychosis case matched by sex and age).*

to play major role". Nevertheless, the relationship between psychosis and offending is described as follows: (a) a direct relationship whereby psychotic symptomology is related to offending (e.g., when hallucinations tell a person to offend); (b) an indirect relationship in which symptomology has some bearing on offending, such as depressive symptoms and irritability, causing the person to act aggressively; and (c) a mediated relationship whereby symptomology is affected by external criminological risk factors, such as alcohol and other drug use, causing an individual to offend [15]. There is evidence that mental health treatment in prison delayed the time to reoffending (18% reduction) following release among individuals with schizophrenia [17].

In this chapter, we present our findings about the association between psychosis and criminal offending (violent and non-violent) in NSW between 2001 and 2015 using data linkage of health and justice administrative data collections. This includes identifying the demographic and criminogenic risk factors for criminal convictions in people with psychosis [1].

Next, we describe the findings from our investigations to examine the impact of two current practices in NSW to reduce reoffending in people with psychosis, namely the court diversion program and utilisation of community mental health services.

Mental health courts, problem-solving courts, court-based diversion programs, and liaison services have been established in response to significant number of individuals with mental illness in the criminal justice system. These programs aim to divert people with mental health issues away from the criminal justice system and into community-based mental health services [18, 19]. Evaluations of such programs, many conducted in the USA, have found positive outcomes in terms of reductions in reoffending, improved social outcomes, and economic benefits [20, 21]. Several studies have also shown cost benefit of such diversion programs [21, 22].

In Australia, court diversion/liaison schemes have expanded over the past two decades [23–26]. In NSW, the Statewide Community and Court Liaison Service (SCCLS) was established in 1999 under the Mental Health [Forensic Provisions] Act to assist magistrates to identify mentally ill offenders charged with less serious criminal offences and provide the option of diverting defendants away from the criminal justice system to in-patient or community psychiatric care [27].

We examined the effectiveness of the SCCLS among individuals with psychosis in NSW between 2001 and 2015 by comparing those receiving a treatment order in the courts with a comparison group receiving punitive sanctions. Specifically, we examined factors associated with the incidence of reoffending, including psychosis type (i.e., schizophrenia and related psychoses, effective psychoses, and substance-related psychoses), offence type (i.e., violent and non-violent offences), socio-demographic factors, and contact with mental health services [14].

We then determined the impact of mental health services contact on reducing reoffending in a 14-year longitudinal study, regardless of receiving a court diversion order. Several studies have demonstrated the impact of antipsychotic medication use on reducing reoffending rates [28–32]. However, medication use represents only one aspect of care for people with psychosis, and these studies have not examined broader health services contacts. For the first time, we investigated the association between contact with mental health services and reoffending in a follow-up study at population level. Using longitudinal linked data, we examined the characteristics of the population of offenders with psychosis in NSW who did not receive a custodial sentence (and thus were at risk of reoffending in the community) during a 14-year follow-up period [13].

For the data linkage, we used de-identified whole-of-population data from New South Wales Ministry' of Health and Justice systems. The linkage study was approved by multiple Ethics Committees, including the NSW Population and Health Services Research Ethics Committee (HREC/15/CIPHS/17), Corrective Services NSW (D15/138715), Cancer Institute NSW (2015/05/586), and the NSW Aboriginal Health and Medical Research Council (1089/15). The linkage study was initially supported by funding from the Mental Health Commission of New South Wales, and more recently Corrective Services NSW.

2. The relationship between psychosis and criminal offending in New South Wales

This section summarises the results from analyses to examine the association between psychosis and criminal offending in New South Wales between 2001 and 2015. We first describe the linked data, followed by an overview of demographic and criminographic characteristics of the psychosis cases and controls. Next, we describe factors associated with criminal conviction, including conviction for violent offences (From Chowdhury et al. 2021 [1]).

2.1 The linked health and offending data

From the NSW Ministry of Health data collections, we obtained the following: psychosis diagnosis type, age at diagnosis, treatment episode start and end date, sex, Aboriginality, marital status, date of birth, and residential area relating to all public and private hospital admissions and presentations to emergency departments in NSW between 2001 and 2012. Codes for psychosis from the International Classification of Diseases (ICD versions 9 and 10) were grouped into three diagnostic types: schizophrenia and related psychoses, affective psychoses, and substance-related psychoses. We used a hierarchical approach to psychosis with those having a diagnosis of schizophrenia and related psychoses coded as "schizophrenia and related psychoses"; any diagnosis of affective psychoses with no diagnosis of schizophrenia and related psychoses was coded as "affective psychoses", and substance-related psychosis in the absence of other two groups was coded as "substance-related psychoses" [16–18]. The index of relative socio-economic disadvantage (IRSD) was used to rank the socio-economic status in each residential area using data on income, education, employment, occupation, and housing [33]. The lowest rank indicates the most disadvantaged areas and the highest rank the most advantaged areas. Residential areas were categorised into disadvantaged (score 1–5) and advantaged (score 6–10).

From the NSW Reoffending Database (RoD), we extracted sex, Aboriginality, offence type, offence date, age at the time of first offence, and principal penalty in the case of court appearance for everyone convicted of a criminal offence. Minor traffic infringements were excluded from the offence data. RoD data were available from 2001 to 2015. Incarceration information was available from the Corrective Services Offender Integrated Management System (OIMS) for all individuals in prison in NSW and the duration of incarceration between 2001 and 2014.

For each case of psychosis, two age- and sex-matched controls without any record of a diagnosis of psychosis were randomly selected from the NSW Ministry of Health data collections that are continuously updated and contain around 178 million records pertaining to more than 15 million individuals [34].

The linked data are presented in **Figure 1**.

2.2 Statistical analysis

Categorical variables were described using frequencies and compared by chi-square tests. Continuous data were presented using means, standard deviations (SD), median, and interquartile ranges (IQRs). Multivariate logistic regression models were used to assess the association between criminal convictions and psychosis, and socio-demographic variables. Associations were determined at the 0.05 level of significance.

2.3 Demographic and criminographic characteristics

Overall, 86,461 individuals (56% men and 44% women) were identified with at least one record of a diagnosis of psychosis, and 172,922 individuals (55.8% men and 44.2% women) were matched by sex and year of birth as controls with no diagnosis of psychosis (**Table 1**).

A comparison of the socio-demographic characteristics of cases with a diagnosis of psychosis and controls showed that psychosis cases were significantly more likely than controls to be from disadvantaged areas than controls (50% *vs.* 42%) and not married (including de facto relationship) (20% *vs.* 36%).

Of a total of 86,461 individuals with psychosis, 26,155 cases (30%) had been convicted of at least one offence during the follow-up period between 2001 and 2015). In comparison, a significantly lower percentage of controls (6%, 10,370 individuals from 172,922) had a criminal conviction during the follow-up period. Violent offences were significantly higher in offenders with psychosis (19%) than controls (3%). About

	Total cases and controls (n = 259,383)		
	Cases (n = 86,461; 33%)	**Controls (n = 172,922; 67%)**	
Variable	n (%)	n (%)	P value
Age groups at most recent diagnosis[1]			<0.001
<20 years	4486 (5)	8085 (4)	
20–29 years	16,456 (19)	31,317 (18)	
30–39 years	19,244 (22)	38,560 (23)	
40+ years	46,275 (54)	94,960 (55)	
Aboriginal			<0.001
Yes	5408 (6)	2531 (2)	
No	80,436 (93)	131,676 (76)	
Unknown	617 (1)	38,715 (22)	
Marital status			<0.001
Married	17,480 (20)	62,102 (36)	
Single	55,832 (65)	44,533 (26)	
Unknown	13,149 (15)	66,287 (38)	
Index of Relative Socio-economic Disadvantage			<0.001
Advantaged	37,628 (44)	74,550 (43)	
Disadvantaged	43,597 (50)	72,989 (42)	
Unknown	5236 (6)	25,383 (15)	
Any criminal conviction			<0.001
Yes	26,155 (30)	10,370 (6)	
No	60,306 (70)	162,552 (94)	
Any violent criminal conviction			<0.001
Yes	16,114 (19)	5156 (3)	
No	70,347 (81)	167,766 (97)	
Any prison episode			<0.001
Yes	9744 (11)	1958 (1)	
No	76,717 (89)	170,964 (99)	

[1]*Recent diagnosis of psychosis for cases and any diagnosis for controls.*

Table 1.
Socio-demographic (2001–2012) and criminographic (2001–2015) characteristics of the cases and controls.

11% of all cases had a prison episode between 2001 and 2014, whereas for controls, this was only 1% (**Table 1**). Those diagnosed with psychosis committed 10% of all offences in NSW between 2001 and 2015. The number of criminal convictions was higher in offenders with substance-related psychoses (median = 3, IQR = 1–6) than those with schizophrenia and related psychoses (median = 2, IQR = 1–5) and affective psychoses (median = 2, IQR = 1–3).

2.3.1 Contact with mental health services

Most records of contact with health services in relation to psychosis were for schizophrenia and related psychoses (82%), followed by affective psychoses (10%) and substance-related psychoses (8%). The median age at first diagnosis for the three psychosis types was: schizophrenia and related psychoses 41 years (IQR = 29–58), affective psychoses 45 years (32–62), and substance-related psychoses 37 years (27–51). However, for those cases convicted of a crime, the median age of first diagnosis across all three diagnosis categories was 31 years (IQR = 24–40).

The median age at first offence for offenders with psychosis and controls was 30 years. This finding suggests that the first-time diagnosis of psychosis in those convicted of a crime occurs after their first offence. It also suggests that the first-time diagnosis of psychosis tends to occur earlier in those who were convicted of a crime than cases with no criminal history.

2.3.2 Criminal convictions in cases and controls

Overall, cases were approximately 5 times more likely than controls to have a criminal conviction (adjusted odds ratio [aOR = 4.68, 95% CI 4.55–4.81). Offence types were similar in offender cases and controls. Twenty-nine per cent of offenders with a diagnosis of psychosis and 31% of offenders with no diagnosis of psychosis had convictions for a violent offence as classified by the Australian and New Zealand Standard of Offence Classification (ANZSOC) [35]. Acts intended to cause injury were the most frequently reported violent offences (23% in cases and controls who offended). Seventy-one per cent of offenders with a diagnosis of psychosis and 69% of offender cases were convicted of non-violent offences. Offences against justice or government procedures (e.g., breaches of custodial orders) were the most commonly reported offences in both cases (17%) and controls (15%), followed by thefts (15% in cases and 12% in controls). Drug offences were 11% in both cases and controls.

Offence types (violent and non-violent) varied by the type of psychosis. Among offenders with a diagnosis of psychosis, violent convictions were more common in those with affective psychoses (34%), followed by schizophrenia and related psychoses (30%), and substance-related psychosis (26%). Non-violent convictions were higher in those with substance-related psychoses (74%), followed by schizophrenia and related psychoses (70%) and affective psychoses (66%).

Sentence types (i.e., non-supervised, supervised, and custodial orders) varied by the type of psychosis. Non-supervised sentences were lowest in those with substance-related psychosis (59% *vs.* 66% in those with schizophrenia and related psychoses and 70% in those with affective psychoses). Those with substance-related psychoses had the highest proportion receiving a custodial sentence (20% *vs.* 17% in those with schizophrenia and related psychoses and 11% in those with affective psychoses).

2.4 Factors associated with criminal convictions

Those with substance-related psychosis had an increased odds of a criminal conviction compared to those with no diagnosis of psychosis (approximately 10 times), followed by schizophrenia and related psychoses (approximately 4 times higher) and affective psychoses (over twice). Those aged between 20 and 39 years had a higher odds of conviction compared with younger age (<20 years). Convictions were approximately

5 times higher in those from Aboriginal backgrounds compared to non-Aboriginal individuals. Convictions were 2 times higher in those who were single than those who were married or in a de facto relationship. Convictions were also significantly more in those from disadvantaged areas when compared with advantaged areas (**Table 2**).

A total of 21,270 cases and controls had at least one conviction for a violent offence, of whom 16,114 (76%) had a diagnosis of psychosis (**Table 1**). Criminal convictions for violence were over 4 times greater in individuals with a diagnosis of psychosis compared to controls (aOR = 4.90, 95% CI 4.73–5.07). Of the cases with a conviction for violence, 74% had a diagnosis of schizophrenia and related psychoses, 20% had a diagnosis of substance-related psychoses, and 6% had a diagnosis of affective psychoses. A gender-stratified analysis showed that men and women with

	Cases and controls (n = 259,383)		
	n (%)	**aOR (95% CI)**	**P value**
Psychosis			
No	172,922 (67)	1	
Yes	86,461 (33)	4.68 (4.55–4.81)	<0.001
Psychosis types			
No psychosis	172,922 (67)	1	
Schizophrenia and related psychoses	65,895 (25)	4.26 (4.13–4.38)	<0.001
Affective psychoses	10,218 (4)	2.49 (2.35–2.65)	<0.001
Substance-related psychoses	10,348 (4)	9.77 (9.32–10.24)	<0.001
Age group			
<20 years	12,571 (5)	1	
20–29 years	47,773 (18)	1.21 (1.15–1.28)	<0.001
30–39 years	57,804 (22)	1.18 (1.12–1.25)	<0.001
40+ years	141,235 (55)	0.37 (0.35–0.39)	<0.001
Marital status			
Married (inc. de facto)	79,582 (31)	1	
Single	100,365 (39)	2.05 (1.98–2.12)	<0.001
Unknown	79,436 (30)	2.32 (2.23–2.42)	<0.001
Aboriginal			
Yes	7939 (3)	5.02 (4.76–5.28)	<0.001
No	212,112 (82)	1	
Unknown	39,332 (15)	0.07 (0.07–0.08)	<0.001
Index of Relative Socio-economic Disadvantage			
Advantaged	112,178 (43)	1	
Disadvantaged	116,586 (45)	1.55 (1.51–1.59)	<0.001
Unknown	30,619 (12)	0.98 (0.93–1.04)	0.521

Table 2.
Adjusted odds ratios (aOR) for at least one criminal conviction (July 2001–June 2015).

a diagnosis of psychosis were more likely to have a conviction for violence compared with men and women without a diagnosis of psychosis. Risk of violent offending was over 4 times in men with psychosis compared with men with no diagnosis of psychosis (aOR = 4.68, 95% CI 4.50–4.87). Among women with psychosis, the risk of violent offending was approximately 9 times higher compared with women with no diagnosis of psychosis (aOR = 8.80, 95% CI 8.01–9.66). This finding reinforces the need to address factors such as gender when designing interventions for specific at-risk groups.

3. The impact of court diversion on reoffending rates in those with psychoses

As described above, a court diversion program has operated in NSW since 1999. The linked data available to the researchers allowed us to conduct an analysis to examine the effectiveness of the program in reducing reoffending among those diagnosed with psychosis by comparing the group diverted to receive treatment (treatment order group) with a comparison group who received a punitive sanction (punitive sanction group) (from Albalawi et al. 2019 [14]). Details of this analysis are published elsewhere [14].

Overall, 7743 individuals with pre-existing diagnoses of psychosis, prior to their court finalisation date for their first principal offence, were identified from the data. We first compared the characteristics of offenders with psychosis, which could influence receiving a treatment order or a punitive sanction order for their first principal offence (i.e., socio-demographic, type of psychosis, and type of offence). We then examined the impact of treatment orders on the incidence of reoffending and time to second offence (reoffending) using the punitive sanction group for comparison in a follow-up period from the court finalisation date for the initial offence to the end of study in 2015. Next, we examined the predictors for the second offence (reoffending) in individuals diagnosed with psychosis.

3.1 Characteristics of the treatment order and comparison (punitive sanction) groups

Of the 7734 individuals with a pre-existing diagnosis of psychosis, 1996 (26%) received treatment order and 5747 (74%) received a punitive sanction for their first principal offence. The punitive sanctions included bonds (47%), fines (44%), suspended sentences (6%), community orders (2%), and probation (<1%).

Between 2001 and 2012, people with psychosis could receive a treatment order in a NSW court where the Statewide Community and Court Liaison Service (SCCLS) was in operation. The SCCLS currently operates in 24 courts across NSW, growing from seven courts in 2001 [36]. We found no significant difference in the proportion of men and women with psychosis who received a treatment order (26% of men and 25% of women). However, we found that a significantly lower proportion of Aboriginal people received a treatment order compared with non-Aboriginal people (19% *vs.* 27%). Court diversion was significantly associated with the type of psychosis, with schizophrenia and related psychoses the most common type of psychosis in the treatment order group with a significantly higher rate compared to the punitive sanction group (81% *vs.* 65%). The most common type of psychosis in the punitive sanction group was substance-related psychoses with a significantly higher rate compared to the treatment order group (25% *vs.* 7%) (**Table 3**).

	Total (N = 7743)		
	Treatment order N = 1996 (26%)	**Punitive sanction** N = 5747 (74%)	*P value*
Age at the first offence			
<18 years	19 (1)	50 (1)	<0.001
18–25 years	393 (20)	1193 (21)	
26–35 years	656 (33)	1979 (34)	
36–45 years	513 (26)	1582 (28)	
46+ years	415 (21)	943 (16)	
Aboriginal			
Yes	148 (7)	625 (11)	<0.001
No	1662 (83)	4514 (79)	
Unknown	186 (9)	608 (11)	
Marital status			
Married	241 (12)	718 (12)	0.625
Other	1755 (88)	5029 (88)	
Country of birth			
Australia	1355 (68)	3988 (69)	<0.001
Other	429 (21)	910 (16)	
Missing	212 (11)	849 (15)	
Psychosis type			
Schizophrenia and related psychoses	1608 (81)	3743 (65)	<0.001
Affective psychosis	241 (12)	555 (10)	
Substance-related psychoses	147 (7)	1449 (25)	
Index of Relative Social Disadvantage			
Advantaged (6–10)	1208 (61)	3065 (53)	<0.001
Disadvantaged (1–5)	788 (39)	1268 (46)	
Type of first offence			
Non-violent offence	873 (44)	3579 (62)	0.457
Violent offence	1123 (56)	2158(38)	

Table 3.
Characteristics of the treatment order and punitive order groups.

Overall, a higher proportion of those with a violent first offence received a treatment order rather than a punitive sanction (56% *vs.* 38%). The most common first principal offence was "Act intended to cause injury", which was significantly higher in the treatment order group than in the punitive sanction group (48% *vs.* 27%). Among those with non-violent first offence, a lower proportion received a treatment order than a punitive sanction (44% *vs.* 62%).

The most common non-violent offence in the diversion group were offences against justice/government procedures (23%), property and environmental damage (22%), and public order (15%), whereas among the punitive sanction group the most common non-violent offence types were drugs (19%), theft (19%), and offences against government procedures (17%).

3.2 Incidence of reoffending in the treatment order and punitive sanction groups

Reoffending (second offence) in the treatment order group was 12% lower than in the punitive sanction group (38% *vs.* 50%) during the follow-up period (i.e., the period between the court finalisation date for the initial offence and the second offence or end of the study). Also, for those who reoffended, the time to second offence was longer in those in the treatment order group. The median number of years from the first offence court finalisation date to the second offence was 5.1 years (IQR = 2.2 – 8.4) in the treatment order group and 4.0 years (IQR = 1.1–1.7) in the punitive sanction group.

The incidence of reoffending in men and women in the treatment order group was lower than in the punitive sanction group. For men, the incidence of reoffending in the treatment order group was 6.8 per 100 person-years and 11.1 per 100 person-years in the punitive sanction group. For women, the incidence of reoffending in the treatment order group was 6.9 per 100 person-years and in the punitive sanction group was 9.6 per 100 person-years. Survival analysis demonstrated a longer time to reoffending for men and women who received treatment orders than those who received punitive sanction over time (see Albalawi et al. [14] for further details [14]).

Analysis of reoffending incidence by type of psychosis showed that diversion order to treatment reduced reoffending, regardless of the type of psychosis. For those with affective psychoses, the incidence of reoffending was 5.3 per 100 person-years in the treatment order group and 7.8 per 100 person-years in the punitive sanction group. For those with schizophrenia and related psychoses, the incidence of reoffering in the treatment order group was 7.0 per 100 person-years and in the punitive sanction group was 10.6 person-years. The incidence of reoffending in those with substance-related psychoses in the treatment order group was 8.1 per 100 person-years and in the punitive sanction group 12.3 per 100 person-years. Time to reoffending was also longer in those who received a treatment order, regardless of type of psychosis. However, survival analysis showed that the treatment orders were least effective in reducing time to reoffending in those with substance-related psychosis ($p = 0.006$) and more effective in reducing reoffending in those with affective psychosis ($p < 0.001$) (details of the survival analysis are given in Albalawi et al. [14]) [14].

Analysis by offence type showed significantly less reoffending in those who received a treatment order than punitive sanction, regardless of the type of first offence (i.e., violent or non-violent). The incidence of reoffending was 7.4 per 100 person-years in individuals who had non-violent first offence and received treatment order. The rate of reoffending for non-violent first offenders was 11.6 per 100 person-years in the punitive sanction group. The incidence of reoffending for the first-time violent offenders who received treatment order was 6.4 per 100 person-years and 9.3 per 100 person-years in the punitive sanction group. Survival analysis demonstrated reduced risk of reoffending in those who received treatment order over time for both violent and non-violent offenders ($p < 0.001$) (**Figure 2**) [14].

3.3 Predictors of reoffending

Cox regression models with random effect were used to identify predictors of reoffending. Analysis was adjusted by age, marital status, country of birth, and psychosis type [14].

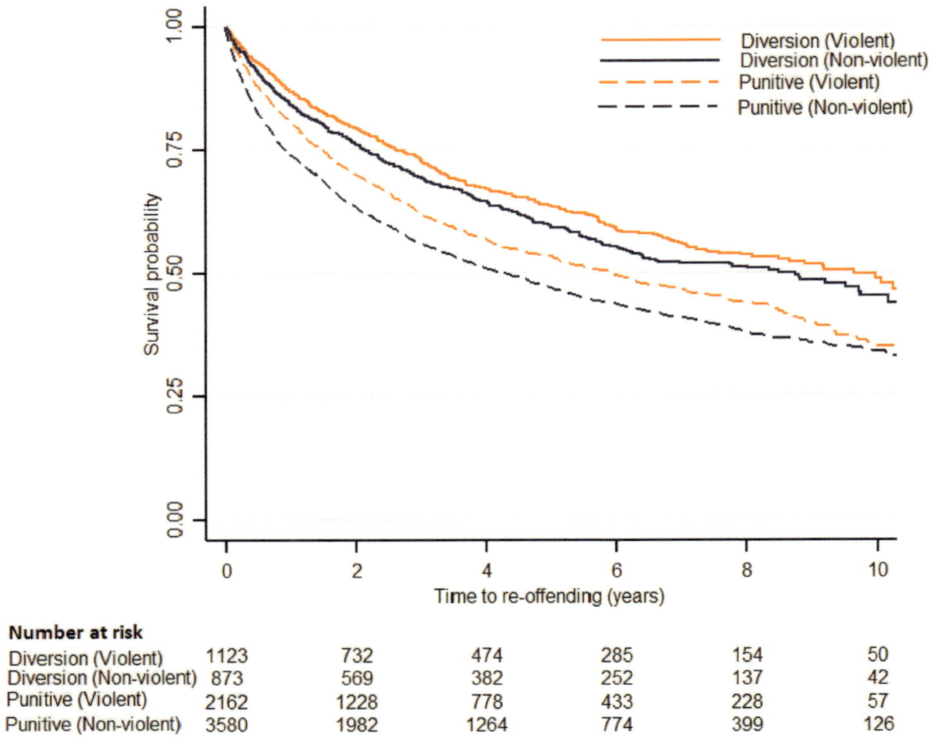

Figure 2.
Kaplan-Meier curves for diversion program versus punitive sanction groups by first principal offence type.

Reoffending was lower in the treatment order group than the punitive sanction group (adjusted hazard ratio [aHR] = 0.68, 95% CI 0.62–0.74). The risk of reoffending varied by type of psychosis. Individuals diagnosed with substance-related psychosis had a higher risk of reoffending than those diagnosed with affective psychoses, regardless of being in the treatment order or punitive sanction group (aHR = 1.46, 95% CI 1.27–1.67). In addition, those who were diagnosed with schizophrenia and related psychoses had a higher risk of reoffending than those with affective psychoses (aHR = 1.19, 95% CI 1.05–1.34). Those whose first offence was non-violent were at a higher risk of reoffending compared to violent offenders (aHR = 1.20, 95 CI 1.12–1.28). Several socio-demographic factors were associated with reoffending. The risk of reoffending was greater in younger age groups and individuals who were not married. Those with an Aboriginal background had an increased risk of reoffending than non-Aboriginal people (aHR = 1.85, 95% CI 1.68–2.03) (**Table A1**) [14].

4. The impact of mental health services utilisation on reoffending rates in those with psychosis

The linked data allowed the first long-term follow-up investigation of the impact of mental health services utilisation on reoffending rates among offenders with psychosis over a 14-year period. This analysis specifically examined clinical contact with mental health services in groups more vulnerable to reoffending. The findings from this analysis inform efforts to enhance mental health services utilisation by people with psychosis who are at higher risk of reoffending (from Adily et al. 2023 [13]).

4.1 Characteristics of the study population

A total of 7393 individuals (70% men and 30% women) received a non-custodial sentence for their first (index) offence following a diagnosis of psychosis between 2001 and 2012. Differences in characteristics of these individuals (socio-demographic, type of psychosis, type of first offence, and contact with mental health services during the follow-up) by gender are summarised in **Table A2**. The most common diagnosis was schizophrenia and related psychoses. A higher proportion of men (69%) were diagnosed with schizophrenia and related psychoses than women (62%). Conversely, women were slightly more than men diagnosed with substance-related psychoses (24% *vs.* 22%) and affective psychoses (14% *vs.* 9%).

While a higher proportion of index offences were non-violent (62%), the most common offences (30%) were violent acts intended to cause injury. Theft was the most frequent non-violent index offence (12.5%). The proportions of violent and non-violent offences were similar among men and women.

Seventy per cent of the study population had at least one mental health service contact during the follow-up period, and slightly higher in women (72%) than men (69%) (**Table A2**). The median number of days from the court finalisation date for the first offence to the first contact with a mental health service was 30 days (IQR: 4–173). The median number of mental health service contacts during the follow-up period was 45 (IQR: 9–171). Most (98%) clinical contacts occurred at community mental health services rather than admission to hospital (1.7%) or emergency department (0.3%). Contact with mental health services was associated with the type of psychosis. Fewer individuals with substance-related psychoses (55%) had contact with mental health services than those with schizophrenia and related psychoses (75%) or affective psychoses (70%). Contact with mental health services was also associated with the type of offence, with more violent offenders having contact than non-violent offenders (74% *vs.* 67%).

4.2 Comparison of reoffending rates in those with mental health service contact and no mental health service contact during the follow-up period

Just less than half of the cohort (49%) reoffended during the follow-up period with over half of second offences (53%) non-violent. The most frequent second offences were acts intended to cause injury (25%). The most common non-violent offences were those against justice procedures, government security, and government operations (18%) (e.g., breach of a community-based order).

Incidence of reoffending among those who had contact with mental health services during the follow-up period (clinical contact group) was lower than those with no clinical contact (7.8 per 100 person-years and 19.1 per 100 person-years, respectively).

Kaplan-Meier survival analysis showed a longer median time to reoffending from the index offence in the clinical contact group (13.56 years) than those who had no mental health service contact during the follow-up (1.69 years). **Figure 3** presents time to reoffending during the follow-up period in those with and without contact with mental health services following their index offence by type of index offence. Time to reoffending was longer for violent offenders who had clinical contact with mental health services during the follow-up period (median survival

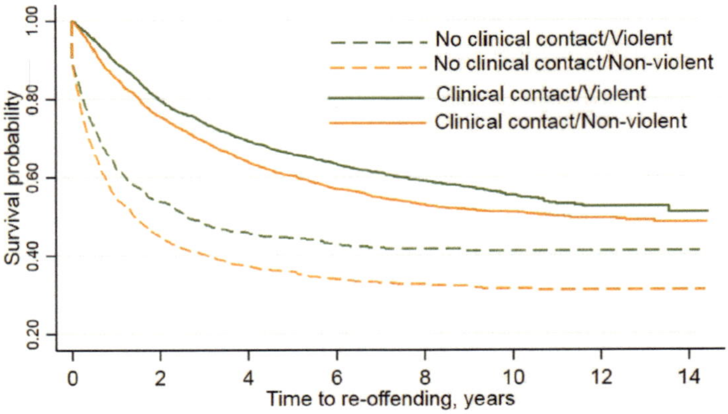

Number at risk								
No clinical contact/Violent	732	386	283	182	109	54	15	2
No clinical contact/Non-violent	1491	654	468	312	203	109	55	4
Clinical contact/Violent	2099	1646	1261	874	556	295	123	10
Clinical contact/Non-violent	3071	2274	1747	1262	860	504	239	34

Figure 3.
Kaplan-Meier plot of time to reoffending in those with and without contact with mental health service following their index offence by type of index offence. The p values of the log-rank are <0.001 in all groups.

time = 12.07 years) compared to violent offenders with no clinical contact (median survival time = 2.59 years). Similarly, time to reoffending was longer for non-violent offenders who had clinical contact with mental health services during the follow-up (median survival time = 10.94 years) than non-violent offenders with no clinical contact with mental health services (median survival time = 1.41 years).

4.3 Risk factors associated with reoffending in men and women

Overall, the risk of reoffending was approximately 55% less in those who had clinical contact with mental health services during the follow-up than those with no clinical contact, regardless of gender (aHR = 0.45, 95% CI 0.42–0.49). Risk of offending was approximately 18% higher in men than women during the follow-up period (aHR = 1.18, 95% CI 1.09–1.27). However, risk of reoffending in men and women who had clinical contact with mental health services during the follow-up was similar. There was a linear relationship between an increased number of clinical contacts and reduced risk of reoffending. Living in a disadvantaged area based on IRSD was not associated with reoffending in men and women. Younger age was associated with reoffending in both men and women with highest risk for those who were less than 18 years of age (**Table A3**).

Our analysis identified gender-specific risk factors for reoffending. Compared to women who were married at the time of index offence, the risk of reoffending was higher for those women who were never married (aHR = 1.25, 95% CI 1.02–1.52) and who had other marital status (e.g., divorced, de facto relationship; aHR = 1.41, 95% CI 1.13–1.74). Aboriginality was another identified gender-specific risk factor for reoffending. Women from Aboriginal background had higher risk of reoffending compared to non-Aboriginal women (aHR = 1.26, 95% CI 1.03–1.53).

Men and women with substance-related psychoses were at higher risk of reoffending compared to men and women with affective psychosis (aHR = 1.27, 95% CI 1.08–1.51 and aHR = 1.30, 95% CI 1.03–1.63, respectively). Both men and women with non-violent index offence were at greater risk of reoffending compared to men and women with violent index offence (aHR = 1.29, 95% CI 1.19–1.40 and aHR = 1.20, 95% CI 1.05–1.38, respectively). A smaller proportion of those with non-violent offences had contact with mental health services than those with violent offences (33% *vs.* 67%, $p < 0.001$).

5. Conclusions

This longitudinal population-based data linkage study examined the association between psychosis and offending, risk factors for offending and reoffending, the impact of court diversion and contact with mental health services on reducing reoffending in individuals diagnosed with psychosis over a 14-year follow-up period (2001–2015). This study specifically focused on identifying the groups at higher risk of reoffending and provided evidence to policymakers, planners, and advocates to develop policies and practices to improve the management of individuals with serious mental illness and prevent contact with the justice system. The outcomes better inform the community about the extent of the problem, pathways leading to contact with the criminal justice system, and promote a better understanding of the needs of those with serious mental illness and ultimately contribute to improved community safety.

While previous studies have focused on the relationship between violence and psychosis [2, 3], the results of this study showed over 4 times higher likelihood of any offending behaviour (violent and non-violent), as determined by proven criminal convictions, in cases with a diagnosis of psychosis compared with age- and sex-matched controls. The likelihood of violent offending in cases with psychosis was 5 times higher than controls [1].

The study showed that the type of psychosis was associated with increased risk of criminal offending with the greater risk for substance-related psychoses, followed by schizophrenia and related psychoses and affective psychoses. Overall, psychosis cases accounted for 10% of all criminal convictions (violent and non-violent) in NSW between 2001 and 2015. Demographic risk factors for offending, regardless of having psychosis, were younger age (20–39 years), living in a disadvantaged area, being unmarried (including de facto relationship), and Aboriginality. These results suggest that interventions targeting the mental health needs of people with psychosis who are at risk of offending are likely to reduce overall rates of offending [1]. We showed that court diversion and contact with mental health services are associated with reduced reoffending. Indeed, we found a linear trend between increased treatment contact and reduced reoffending [13, 14, 37].

The results from our study suggest that most offenders with psychosis were diagnosed following offending. The median age at first criminal conviction in people with psychosis was 30 years, and the median age at first diagnosis of psychosis was 31 years [1]. These results are consistent with a Western Australian study where the first arrest in those with a psychiatric illness preceded the first contact with mental health services [38]. This suggests that policies for the early detection of psychosis are appropriate to improve health and justice outcomes. The challenges in early detection and avoidance of contact with mental health services by patients are acknowledged. In our data, the median age at first diagnosis for cases diagnosed with affective psychoses and schizophrenia and related psychoses was 45 and 41 years, respectively. Cases with substance-related psychoses were diagnosed earlier (median age = 33 years), which may be related to more frequent contact with health services due to adverse health outcomes of substance use.

Substance-related psychoses were more frequent in those who have been convicted for offences and reinforces the well-established link between drug use and offending, most likely as a result of committing acquisitive crimes to fund problem drug use [38]. As we used a hierarchical approach to categorise diagnoses, this suggests that substance-related psychoses alone makes a significant contribution to criminal convictions. However, we found lower prevalence of violent convictions in this group compared with those with schizophrenia and related psychoses and affective psychoses.

At the time of the study, Aboriginal people accounted for 3% of the total NSW population [39]. However, we found that Aboriginal people were 5 times more likely to be convicted of a crime than non-Aboriginal people. We also found that 6% of cases with a diagnosis of psychoses in our data were Aboriginal [1]. These findings raise questions about the availability and nature of treatment options and engagement of Aboriginal people with mental health services. This suggests further investigation of cultural appropriateness of mental health services for Aboriginal people who may be at risk of offending to ensure they receive equitable treatment. Our analysis showed a concerning trend that Aboriginal people were significantly less likely to be diverted into treatment by the courts than non-Aboriginal people (19% *vs.* 27%) [14, 40].

Our linkage study allowed us to undertake the most comprehensive evaluation of a court diversion program for those with a serious mental illness (psychosis) in Australia. Our findings have shown that the overall risk of reoffending was 32% lower in those who received treatment orders, regardless of offence type (violent or non-violent) than those who received a punitive sanction, such as a fine, community order, or good behaviour bond. In addition, we found that time to subsequent reoffending was significantly longer for those who received treatment orders than those who received punitive sanctions (5.1 *vs.* 4.0 years, respectively). The number of treatment episodes was also associated with a reduced hazard of offending. Taken together, these three findings provide compelling evidence of the role of engagement with mental health services, and the diversion by the courts into mental health services, as an important strategy to reduce offending in this group.

The study provides potential insights into magistrates' sentencing patterns for different offender groups. Overall, almost three-quarters of those with a prior diagnosis of psychosis were given punitive sanctions rather than a treatment order. The reasons for this are unclear. It may suggest caution on the part of magistrates to divert those before the courts into mental health services, a lack of awareness of, and confidence in the evidence of effectiveness of treatment and engagement with mental health services, or a lack of awareness of a history of psychosis in those appearing in court. Diversion into treatment is discretionary and magistrates are not obliged to order mental health treatment, even if the expert evidence is available to support the presence of a mental illness/condition or developmental disability [41]. In addition, legal decision-making involves a different set of criteria that influence outcomes from a legal perspective as compared to a medical perspective. In NSW, court diversion is only available to those who are charged with minor offences and appear at the local Magistrate's courts when the process of prosecution has begun (i.e., pre-trial) [24]. The individuals who are already being treated by mental health services may not receive a treatment order. In addition, magistrates have the option of ordering a conditional bond that could include the expectation to pursue mental health treatment [14].

After determining mental illness/condition or developmental disability, the magistrate considers several factors, including seriousness of the offence, the association of offence with mental illness/condition or disability, the existing treatment/management plan, and likelihood of adherence to treatment/management plan in their decision to divert an individual away from the criminal justice system and into treatment. The magistrates need to balance legal issues such as the need for punishment and deterrence, with public interests in diverting a particular individual into treatment.

The very low diversion rate (26%) for those with a history of psychosis may reflect the complexity of this decision-making process. For example, a low confidence of magistrates in the individuals' potential to adhere to the treatment plan and responsible mental health services willingness to notify the court about the treatment breaches by the treating clinicians [14]. It may also represent a lack of awareness by lawyers of the effectiveness of the mental health diversion process in reducing subsequent offending or a lack of awareness of their client's mental health history. Publicly funded lawyers and the courts are often under intense pressure to resolve cases as quickly as possible and so there may be a reluctance to delay matters while the person is referred for mental health assessment. More research is needed into this, such that equitable access to diversion exists.

Our investigation of sentencing patterns has shown that those who had a diagnosis of psychosis closer to the time of the court finalisation date were more likely to receive a treatment order than those with a more remote diagnosis. This may be related to the magistrate's awareness of the status of mental illness and its relation to a history of offending behaviour of the individual, which could lead to their decision to hand down a punitive sanction. On the other hand, closer proximity between the diagnosis of psychosis and the court appearance may prompt the magistrate to order treatment to prevent future offending by the individual. However, this could also reflect the effectiveness of having an on-site court liaison service available to the court to provide a more immediate opinion and increase confidence in a forensic mental health opinion, given the pressure on magistrates to finalise matters and clear court backlogs [14]. It is possible that a treatment order is a means of disposing of cases quickly. In 2017, the NSW government invested AU$39 million dollars to appoint new judges to clear court backlogs in NSW [42]. In addition, it has been found that the odds of diversion were 10 times higher for those with legal representation than those without. This finding reinforces the importance of affording legal representation for individuals with serious mental illness [40].

While the expectation was to see more punitive sanction orders for individuals with more serious offences, those with violent offences were more likely to be diverted into treatment rather than receiving a punitive sanction [40]. It is possible that magistrates regard the violent behaviour as being more likely driven by the psychosis and thus mitigating the level of responsibility [14]. However, the data suggest that those with substance-related psychoses were less likely to be diverted than those with affective psychoses or schizophrenia or related psychosis, regardless of type of offence (violent or non-violent). This may reflect the strong association between substance use and reoffending and a view by magistrates that substance use is an intractable problem [14].

We examined the impact of clinical contact with mental health services on the risk of reoffending in people with psychosis. The follow-up period for this analysis ranged from 2.5 to 14 years from the initial offence. This analysis shows that most of the cohort (70%) had clinical contacts following their initial offence and most contacts (98%) occurred at community mental health services rather than emergency rooms or hospital admissions. It is acknowledged that the data did not include the clinical mental health services provided by general practitioners or private clinicians. The median number of clinical contacts during the follow-up period was 45 times. Half of the first contacts with a mental health service occurred within 30 days and 75% occurred within 6 months following the court finalisation date for the initial offence [13]. Our 2-year follow-up analysis of the data found that increased early contact with community mental health services (i.e., within

30 days from court finalisation date for the initial offence) reduced the risk of reoffending in male offenders with psychoses [37].

Almost one-third of the cohort had no contact with mental health services. On average, the risk of reoffending was more than twice in those without contact with mental health services during the follow-up period compared to those who utilised mental health services. The risk of reoffending was reduced by an increased number of contacts with mental health services. Those with no clinical contact had more than a fivefold risk of reoffending compared to those with the highest number of contacts. Of those who offended, the time to reoffend was 12 months longer in those who had contact with mental health services than those with no contact, regardless of type of psychosis or offence highlighting the importance of treatment in the prevention of reoffending.

Individuals with substance-related psychoses tended to have fewer clinical contacts with mental health services compared to other types of psychosis. However, it is acknowledged that those with substance-related psychoses may have had clinical contact with other health practitioners during the course of treatment for drug related issues. Additionally, those with non-violent initial offences had less contact with mental health services than those who committed violent offences. Both substance-related psychoses and non-violent offending were found to be the risk factors for reoffending.

Earlier, we discussed the magistrates' sentencing patterns, noting fewer treatment orders for individuals with substance-related psychoses and non-violent offences. Other identified risk factors for reoffending were younger age, not being married, and Aboriginality. In our cohort, we specifically found higher rate of reoffending in Aboriginal women compared with non-Aboriginal women. Overall, there was higher risk of reoffending in men than women. These findings highlight the necessity of improving follow-up plans to address demographic and criminological risk factors for reoffending. This includes providing better access to diversion programs, general practice, and both public and private mental health services. Additionally, further investigation is underway to assess the need for other support services, such as housing.

The findings from this body of work informed an investigation to identify and describe the key attributes of an "optimal model of care" using a Delphi model and involving experts and consumers [43]. The outcomes of this process are now being integrated into a multidisciplinary transition care plan for individuals with psychosis exiting prison in NSW. This plan engages multiple agencies, including community mental health services, drug and alcohol services, and general practitioners, with the aim of preventing reoffending and improving health, welfare, and justice outcomes for the vulnerable and at-risk groups with serious mental illness [44].

Acknowledgements

All authors of the original papers that are summarised in this chapter [1, 13, 14] are acknowledged, specifically Assistant Professor Olayan Albalawi and Dr. Nabila Chowdhury who performed data analysis; A/Professor Handan Wand and Dr. Azar Kariminia for provision of data analysis and reporting; Professor Peter Schofield, Professor Grant Sara, and Professor David Greenberg for their clinical advice, and Mr. Luke Grant, Deputy Commissioner of Corrective Services NSW, for his contributions to facilitate financial support and input on manuscripts arising from the study. The authors acknowledge the Centre for Health Record Linkage (CheReL) from the NSW Ministry of Health for data linkage. The study was funded by the Mental Health Commission of New South Wales and Corrective Services NSW.

Conflict of interest

The authors declare no conflict of interest.

Appendices and nomenclature

	Total (N = 7743)		
	N (%)	**aHR (95 CI)**	**p-value**
Group			
Punitive sanction	1571 (75)	1	
Diversion program	529 (25)	0.68 (0.62–0.74)	<0.001
Psychosis type			
Mood disorder with psychosis	265 (13)	1	
Schizophrenia and delusional disorder	1387 (66)	1.19(1.05–1.34)	0.005
Psychosis due to psychoactive substance use	448 (21)	1.46(1.27–1.67)	<0.001
Age at the first offence			
<18 years	37 (2)	2.26(1.65–3.09)	<0.001
18–25 years	400 (19)	1.57(1.40–1.77)	<0.001
26–35 years	701 (33)	1.64(1.47–1.83)	<0.001
36–45 years	592 (28)	1.34(1.19–1.50)	<0.001
46+ years	370 (18)	1	
Aboriginal			
No	1526 (73)	1	
Yes	299 (14)	1.85(1.68–2.03)	<0.001
Unknown	275 (13)	0.08(0.06–0.11)	<0.001
Marital status			
Married	344 (16)	1	
Other	1756 (84)	1.21(1.09–1.35)	<0.001
Country of birth			
Other	320 (18)	1	
Australia	1493 (71)	1.18(1.08–1.30)	<0.001
Unknown	287 (14)	1.27(1.12–1.45)	<0.001
First principal offence type			
Violent	2399 (43)	1	
Non-violent	3244 (57)	1.20(1.12–1.28)	<0.001

[a]*Adjusted by age, marital status, country of birth, and psychosis type.*

Table A1.
Adjusted hazard ratios (aHRs) for reoffending[a].

Characteristics	Total N = 7393	Male N = 5208 (70%)	Female N = 2185 (30%)	p-value
Age group at index offence				**<0.001**
<18 years	212 (3)	119 (2)	93 (4)	
18–25 years	1423 (19)	1019 (20)	404 (19)	
26–35 years	2440 (33)	1753 (34)	687 (31)	
36–45 years	2021 (27)	1404 (30)	617 (28)	
46+ years	1297 (18)	913 (18)	384 (18)	
Aboriginal				**<0.001**
No	5737 (78)	4154 (80)	1583 (72)	
Yes	487 (7)	277 (5)	210 (10)	
Unknown	1169 (16)	777 (15)	392 (18)	
Marital status				**<0.001**
Married	903 (12)	533 (10)	370 (17)	
Never married	4258 (58)	3172 (61)	1086 (50)	
Other	2232 (30)	1503 (29)	729 (33)	
Country of birth				**0.024**
Other	1172 (16)	863 (17)	309 (14)	
Australia	5290 (71)	3705 (71)	1585 (73)	
Missing	931 (13)	640 (12)	291 (13)	
IRSD[1]				0.134
Advantaged (6–10)	2885 (39)	2061 (40)	824 (38)	
Disadvantaged (1–5)	4508 (61)	3147 (60)	1361 (62)	
Type of psychosis				**<0.001**
Affective psychoses	780 (11)	466 (9)	314 (14)	
Schizophrenia and related psychoses	4967 (67)	3616 (69)	1351 (62)	
Substance-related psychoses	1646 (22)	1126 (22)	520 (24)	
Type of index offence				0.863
Non-violent	4562 (62)	3217 (62)	1345 (62)	
Violent	2831 (38)	1991 (38)	840 (38)	
Contact with mental health services during the follow-up period				**0.009**
No	2223 (30)	1613 (31)	610 (28)	
Yes	5170 (70)	3595 (69)	1575 (72)	
Number of contacts with mental health services during the follow-up period				**0.005**
0	2223 (30)	1613 (31)	610 (28)	
1–5	1001 (14)	722 (14)	279 (13)	
6–20	955 (13)	684 (13)	271 (12)	
21–60	921 (12)	616 (12)	305 (14)	
61–200	1146 (15)	777 (15)	369 (17)	
≥201	1147 (16)	796 (15)	351 (16)	

[1]*IRSD: Index of Relative Socioeconomic Disadvantage.*

Table A2.
Baseline characteristics of the study population and their contact with mental health services during the follow-up period by gender.

	Total			Men			Women		
Characteristics	**Reoffending n (%)**	**aHR (95% CI)**	**p**	**Reoffending n (%)**	**aHR (95% CI)**	**p**	**Reoffending n (%)**	**aHR (95% CI)**	**p**
Gender				—	—	—	—	—	—
Female	968 (27)	1		—	—	—	—	—	—
Male	2627 (73)	1.18 (1.09–1.27)	**<0.001**	—	—	—	—	—	—
Age at index offence									
<18 years	135 (4)	2.35 (1.93–2.86)	**<0.001**	82 (3)	2.49 (1.95–3.19)	**<0.001**	53 (5)	2.18 (1.56–3.05)	**<0.001**
18–25 years	804 (22)	1.78 (1.57–2.01)	**<0.001**	588 (22)	1.76 (1.53–2.03)	**<0.001**	216 (22)	1.85 (1.46–2.35)	**<0.001**
26–35 years	1323 (37)	1.72 (1.54–1.92)	**<0.001**	979 (37)	1.73 (1.51–1.96)	**<0.001**	344 (36)	1.74 (1.39–2.16)	**<0.001**
36–45 years	900 (25)	1.34 (1.19–1.50)	**<0.001**	660 (25)	1.37 (1.20–1.57)	**<0.001**	240 (25)	1.28 (1.02–1.61)	**0.030**
46+ years	433 (12)	1		318 (12)	1		115 (12)	1	
Aboriginal									
No	2822 (78)	1		2123 (81)	1		699 (72)	1	
Yes	275 (8)	1.20 (1.05–1.36)	**0.005**	156 (6)	1.15 (0.97–1.35)	0.099	119 (12)	1.26 (1.03–1.53)	**0.026**
Unknown	498 (14)	0.78 (0.71–0.86)	**<0.001**	348 (13)	0.78 (0.69–0.87)	**<0.001**	150 (15)	0.80 (0.67–0.95)	**0.013**
Marital status									
Married	360 (10)	1		231 (9)	1		129 (13)	1	

	Total			Men			Women		
Characteristics	**Reoffending n (%)**	**aHR (95% CI)**	**p**	**Reoffending n (%)**	**aHR (95% CI)**	**p**	**Reoffending n (%)**	**aHR (95% CI)**	**p**
Never married	2201 (61)	1.17 (1.04–1.31)	**0.009**	1687 (64)	1.11 (0.97–1.28)	0.136	514 (53)	1.25 (1.02–1.52)	**0.030**
Other	1034 (29)	1.19 (1.04–1.36)	**0.009**	709 (27)	1.09 (0.93–1.28)	0.299	325 (34)	1.41 (1.13–1.74)	**0.002**
Country of birth									
Other	546 (15)	1		426(16)	1		120 (12)	1	
Australia	2618 (73)	0.99 (0.90–1.09)	0.854	1902 (73)	0.96 (0.86–1.07)	0.479	716 (74)	1.09 (0.90–1.34)	0.378
Missing	431 (12)	0.94 (0.81–1.09)	0.405	299 (11)	0.93 (0.78–1.10)	0.393	132 (14)	0.99 (0.75–1.31)	0.945
IRSD									
Advantaged (6–10)	1394 (39)	1		1036 (39)	1		358 (37)	1	
Disadvantaged (1–5)	2201 (61)	1.02 (0.95–1.09)	0.649	1591 (61)	1.02 (0.94–1.1)	0.674	610 (63)	1.00 (0.88–1.15)	0.942
Type of psychosis									
Affective psychoses	326 (9)	1		205 (8)	1		121 (13)	1	
Schizophrenia and related psychoses	2401 (67)	1.12 (1.00–1.26)	0.060	1813 (69)	1.11 (0.96–1.29)	0.153	588 (61)	1.13 (0.93–1.38)	0.231
Substance-related psychoses	868 (24)	1.29 (1.13–1.47)	**<0.001**	609 (23)	1.27 (1.08–1.51)	**0.003**	259 (27)	1.30 (1.03–1.63)	**0.025**
Type of index offence									
Violent	2362 (66)	1		1733 (66)	1		629 (65)	1	

Characteristics	Total			Men			Women		
	Reoffending n (%)	**aHR (95% CI)**	**p**	**Reoffending n (%)**	**aHR (95% CI)**	**p**	**Reoffending n (%)**	**aHR (95% CI)**	**p**
Non-violent	1233 (34)	1.26 (1.18–1.35)	**<0.001**	894 (34)	1.29 (1.19–1.40)	**<0.001**	339 (35)	1.20 (1.05–1.38)	**0.006**
Contact with mental health services									
No	1394 (39)	1		1036 (39)	1		358 (37)	1	
Yes	2201 (61)	0.45 (0.42–0.49)	**<0.001**	1591 (61)	0.45 (0.42–0.49)	**<0.001**	610 (63)	0.46 (0.40–0.52)	**<0.001**
Number of contacts with mental health services									
0	1394 (39)	5.78 (5.04–6.62)	**<0.001**	1036 (39)	5.77 (4.92–6.77)	**<0.001**	358 (37)	5.95 (4.55–7.78)	**<0.001**
1–5	599 (17)	4.59 (3.95–5.32)	**<0.001**	438 (17)	4.48 (3.77–5.33)	**<0.001**	161 (17)	5.01 (3.75–6.70)	**<0.001**
6–20	513 (14)	3.76 (3.23–4.38)	**<0.001**	378 (14)	3.75 (3.14–4.48)	**<0.001**	135 (14)	3.87 (2.87–5.21)	**<0.001**
21–60	409 (11)	2.79 (2.38–3.26)	**<0.001**	283 (11)	2.73 (2.27–3.29)	**<0.001**	126 (13)	3.00 (2.22–4.06)	**<0.001**
61–200	430 (12)	2.12 (1.82–2.48)	**<0.001**	307 (12)	2.12 (1.77–2.55)	**<0.001**	123 (13)	2.16 (1.60–2.92)	**<0.001**
≥201	250 (7)	1		185 (7)	1		65 (7)	1	

Table A3.
Adjusted hazard ratios for reoffending during the follow-up period.

Author details

Armita Adily[1*], Stephen Allnutt[2] and Tony Butler[3]

1 School of Population Health, UNSW Sydney, Sydney, Australia

2 School of Psychiatry, UNSW Sydney, Sydney, Australia

3 Justice Health Research Program, School of Population Health, UNSW Sydney, Sydney, Australia

*Address all correspondence to: a.adily@unsw.edu.au

References

[1] Chowdhury NZ et al. Psychosis and criminal offending: A population-based data-linkage study. Criminal Justice and Behaviour. 2021;**48**(2):0093854820964834

[2] Douglas KS, Guy LS, Hart SD. Psychosis as a risk factor for violence to others: A meta-analysis. Psychological Bulletin. 2009;**135**(5):679-706

[3] Fazel S et al. Schizophrenia and violence: Systematic review and meta-analysis. PLoS Medicine. 2009;**6**(8):e1000120

[4] Fazel S, Yu R. Psychotic disorders and repeat offending: Systematic review and meta-analysis. Schizophrenia Bulletin. 2011;**37**(4):800-810

[5] Steadman HJ et al. Prevalence of serious mental illness among jail inmates. Psychiatric Services. 2009;**60**(6):761-765

[6] Nielssen O et al. Outcome of serious violent offenders with psychotic illness and cognitive disorder dealt with by the New South Wales criminal justice system. The Australian and New Zealand Journal of Psychiatry. 2019;**53**(5):441-446

[7] Fazel S, Grann M. The population impact of severe mental illness on violent crime. The American Journal of Psychiatry. 2006;**163**(8):1397-1403

[8] SCRGSP (Steering Committee for the Review of Government Service Provision) 2024, Report on Government Services 2024, Productivity Commission, Canberra. Available from: https://www.pc.gov.au/ongoing/report-on-government-services/2024/data-downloads/rogs-2024-partc-overview-and-sections.pdf. ISSN 2205-5703

[9] Shea P. Mullen, Paul (2001) A review of the relationship between mental disorders and offending Behaviours and on the management of mentally abnormal offenders in the health and criminal justice services. Current Issues in Criminal Justice. 2002;**13**(3):344-345

[10] Mullen PE. Schizophrenia and violence: From correlations to preventive strategies. Advances in Psychiatric Treatment. 2006;**12**(4):239-248

[11] Payne J. Recidivism in Australia: Findings and Future Research. Canberra: Australian Institute of Criminology; 2007

[12] Australian Bureau of Statistics. (Sep - quarter -2024). Corrective Services, Australia. ABS. Available from: https://www.abs.gov.au/statistics/people/crime-and-justice/corrective-services-australia/sep-quarter-2024

[13] Adily A et al. Mental health service utilisation and reoffending in offenders with a diagnosis of psychosis receiving non-custodial sentences: A 14-year follow-up study. The Australian and New Zealand Journal of Psychiatry. 2023;**57**(3):411-422

[14] Albalawi O et al. Court diversion for those with psychosis and its impact on re-offending rates: Results from a longitudinal data-linkage study. BJPsych Open. 2019;**5**(1):e9

[15] Peterson JK et al. How often and how consistently do symptoms directly precede criminal behavior among offenders with mental illness? Law and Human Behavior. 2014;**38**(5):439-449

[16] Bonta J, Blais J, Wilson HA. A theoretically informed meta-analysis

of the risk for general and violent recidivism for mentally disordered offenders. Aggression and Violent Behavior. 2014;**19**(3):278-287

[17] Igoumenou A, Kallis C, Coid J. Treatment of psychosis in prisons and violent recidivism. BJPsych open. 2015;**1**(2):149-157

[18] Schneider RD. Mental health courts and diversion programs: A global survey. International Journal of Law and Psychiatry. 2010;**33**(4):201-206

[19] Richardson E, McSherry B. Diversion down under—Programs for offenders with mental illnesses in Australia. International Journal of Law and Psychiatry. 2010;**33**(4):249-257

[20] Steadman HJ, Naples M. Assessing the effectiveness of jail diversion programs for persons with serious mental illness and co-occurring substance use disorders. Behavioral Sciences & the Law. 2005;**23**(2):163-170

[21] Skrzypiec G, Wundersitz J, McRostie H. Magistrates Court Diversion Program: An Analysis of Post-Program Offending. Adelaide: Government of South Australia, Office of Crime Statistics and Research; 2004. Available from: https://catalogue.nla.gov.au/catalog/3371010

[22] Hughes D. A simulation modeling approach for planning and costing jail diversion programs for persons with mental illness. In: Taxman FS, Pattavina A, editors. Simulation Strategies to Reduce Recidivism: Risk Need Responsivity (RNR) Modeling for the Criminal Justice System. New York, NY: Springer; 2013. pp. 223-265

[23] Steadman HJ, Morris SM, Dennis DL. The diversion of mentally ill persons from jails to community-based services: A profile of programs. American Journal of Public Health. 1995;**85**(12):1630-1635

[24] Greenberg D, Nielsen B. Court diversion in NSW for people with mental health problems and disorders. NSW Public Health Bulletin. 2002;**13**(7):158-160

[25] James DV. Court diversion in perspective. The Australian and New Zealand Journal of Psychiatry. 2006;**40**(6-7):529-538

[26] Davidson F et al. A critical review of mental health court liaison services in Australia: A first national survey. Psychiatry, Psychology and Law. 2016;**23**(6):908-921

[27] Bradford D. An evaluation of the NSW court liaison services. In: Smith NE, editor. NSW Bureau of Crime Statistics and Research. Sydney: Attorney General's Department of NSW; 2009

[28] Baruch N et al. An evaluation of the use of olanzapine pamoate depot injection in seriously violent men with schizophrenia in a UK high-security hospital. Therapeutic Advances in Psychopharmacology. 2014;**4**(5):186-192

[29] Fazel S et al. Antipsychotics, mood stabilisers, and risk of violent crime. The Lancet. 2014;**384**(9949):1206-1214

[30] Kasinathan J, Sharp G, Barker A. Evaluation of olanzapine pamoate depot in seriously violent males with schizophrenia in the community. Therapeutic Advances in Psychopharmacology. 2016;**6**(5):301-307

[31] Mohr P et al. Long-acting injectable antipsychotics for prevention and management of violent behaviour in psychotic patients. International Journal of Clinical Practice. 2017;**71**(9):e12997, 1-7

[32] Rezansoff SN et al. Adherence to antipsychotic medication and criminal recidivism in a Canadian provincial offender population. Schizophrenia Bulletin. 2017;**43**(5):1002-1010

[33] Australian Bureau of Statistics. Census of Population and Housing: Socio-Economic Indexes for Areas (SEIFA), Australia, 2011. Australian Bureau of Statistics; 2023. Available from: https://www.abs.gov.au/ausstats/abs@.nsf/Lookup/2033.0.55.001main+features100052011

[34] Centre for Health Record Linkage. CHeReL Master Linkage Key. 2024. Available from: https://www.cherel.org.au/datasets

[35] Australian Bureau of Statistics. Australian and New Zealand Standard Offence Classification (ANZSOC). ABS; 2011. Available from: https://www.abs.gov.au/statistics/classifications/australian-and-new-zealand-standard-offence-classification-anzsoc/latest-release

[36] Mental health commission of New South Wales. Statewide community and Court Liaison Service (SCCLS). 2023. Available from: https://www.nswmentalhealthcommission.com.au/content/statewide-community-and-court-liaison-service-sccls

[37] Adily A et al. Association between early contact with mental health services after an offense and reoffending in individuals diagnosed with psychosis. JAMA Psychiatry. 2020;**77**(11):1-10

[38] Morgan VA et al. A whole-of-population study of the prevalence and patterns of criminal offending in people with schizophrenia and other mental illness. Psychological Medicine. 2013;**43**(9):1869-1880

[39] Australian Bureau of Statistics. 2071.0—Census of Population and Housing: Reflecting Australia—Stories from the Census, 2016. Canberra: Australian Bureau of Statistics; 2018

[40] Macdonald C et al. Who gets diverted into treatment? A study of defendants with psychosis. Psychiatry, Psychology and Law. 2024;**31**(1):132-145

[41] Howard D, Westmore B. Crime and Mental Health Law in New South Wales: A Practical Guide for Lawyers and Health Care Professionals. 3rd ed. Chatswood: LexisNexis Butterworths; 2018

[42] Ingall J. New Judges to Tackle Regional Court Backlog. 2017. Available from: https://www.abc.net.au/news/2017-07-24/district-court-judges-tackle-case-backlog-regional-nsw/8738006

[43] Simpson PL et al. Defining optimal post-prison care for those with psychosis: A Delphi study. Frontiers in Psychiatry. 2021;**12**:760904

[44] Justice Health and Forensic Mental Health Network. Community Transitions Trial Service Model—Community Forensic Mental Health. July 2020–June 2021. Sydney: Justice Health and Forensic Mental Health Network; 2020

Section 5

Social and Global Perspectives

Chapter 10

Perspective Chapter: The Interplay of Stigma and Psychosis

Sunday Oritsetimenyin Otimenyin and Esther Badugu Patrick

Abstract

Stigma significantly impacts individuals with psychosis, exacerbating their symptoms and hindering recovery. This review explores the complex relationship between stigma and psychosis, highlighting how societal attitudes and misconceptions about mental illness contribute to the problem. Stigma arises from various sources, including lack of understanding, misinformation, historical and cultural factors, media portrayals, social and economic factors, and personal experiences. It worsens psychotic symptoms by promoting stress, anxiety, social isolation, and non-adherence to treatment, and it increases the risk of suicide, delays treatment, and reduces the quality of life for those affected. Effective management of stigma involves education, advocacy, and supportive interventions. Counseling is a key tool, helping to build self-esteem, enhance self-worth, and challenge negative self-talk. Technological advancements such as telehealth, mobile apps, online platforms, virtual reality therapy, mindfulness and meditation apps, and deep brain stimulation also contribute to stigma management. Understanding the multifaceted impact of stigma on psychosis and other mental health illnesses is crucial for improving outcomes and providing holistic care for affected individuals. Promoting stigma awareness and empowering individuals with psychosis to live fulfilling lives are essential steps toward creating a more inclusive society.

Keywords: psychosis, mental health, suicide, depression, stigma, telehealth

1. Introduction

Mental health is an important and a critical component of overall well-being of humans and animals. Mental health comprises how we think, feel, and act in everyday life. A supposed person with sound mental health is expected to think, feel, and act according to what is stipulated as normal behaviors. Deviation from the normal is classified as having a mental health issue. Conscious efforts are made to ensure that humans operate within normal behaviors. Just as we take steps to protect our physical health, it is important to prioritize mental health, seek support when needed, and build environments that promote emotional and psychological well-being. Efforts to improve mental health awareness, reduce stigma, and ensure access to care will foster healthier, more resilient individuals and communities and ensure a safer environment [1].

Mental health challenges are common in societies and communities. The fraction of society that has mental illnesses negatively impacts the society with impact on: man hour loss and economic impact, family suffering and safety concerns, and insurgencies and security of society. A percentage of the society has mental health challenges; this percentage, though small, poses a great challenge to society. Mental health challenges are characterized by abnormal, harmful, resentful, and unusual behaviors, generally classified as abnormal behaviors. These behaviors are not acceptable to the general public, family members, and sometimes to the person who is plagued. There is a tendency to withdraw or dissociate from anyone with these health challenges, for fear of being maltreated by the person. Withdrawal leads to stigmatizing the patients and isolating them from society. Unfortunately, such actions worsen the predicaments of the patient. It can plunge them into depression or drive them to commit suicide or make them to be violent and harmful to themselves and society. The care of mentally derailed patient must be a joint and collaborative effort of society. This is necessary for sound economic growth and the safety of society and its environment. Urgent awareness in communities enables members of the communities to rise to their responsibilities.

There is a complex relationship between stigma and psychosis [2]. Exploring how societal attitudes and misconceptions surrounding mental illness can significantly impact the lives of individuals experiencing psychotic episodes is necessary. There is a multifaceted nature of stigma, its origins, and its far-reaching consequences for individuals with psychosis. Stigma plays a major role in exacerbating the symptoms of psychosis and hindering recovery [3]. The intricate dynamics between these two phenomena, if well understood, can lead to the development of strategies to reduce stigma and improve the lives of patients affected by psychosis and related mental illness.

1.1 Factors that cause/predispose to psychosis

A number of factors could predispose to psychosis or worsen psychosis:

1. Stigmatization of psychotic patients or those predisposed to psychosis.
2. Family history of psychosis
3. Possession of genes linked to psychosis
4. Stressful life events
5. Substance abuse
6. Infections that lead to brain damage
7. Age
8. Social factors [4, 5]

1.2 Stigma and its impact

Stigma remains a significant barrier to recovery of individuals with psychosis/mental illness. Stigma may predispose prone persons to psychosis. Understanding the origins and consequences of stigma promotes works/actions that reduce its impact on psychosis and create a more inclusive society. Awareness is promoted through education, advocacy, and supportive interventions. Individuals with psychosis should be empowered to live a fulfilling life and reach their full potential. Stigma and the process of stigmatization consist of two fundamental elements: recognition of the differentiating "mark" and the subsequent devaluation of the person [5]; capitalizing on the person's shortcomings and exposing the person's weaknesses to the general public.

2. Definition of psychosis and stigma

Psychosis: Psychosis is a mental health condition characterized by a disconnection from reality and societal values. Symptoms of psychosis include: hallucinations, delusions, disorganized thinking, and altered behavior. The causative factors of psychosis are not well understood, but it can be caused by various factors, including mental illness, substance abuse, and an adverse condition that strains mental capabilities (bereavement, mishaps) or medical conditions.

Stigma: Stigma often results from mark of societal disapproval. Stigma and the process of stigmatization consist of two fundamental elements, the recognition of the differentiating "mark" and the subsequent devaluation of the person [5]. It is a mark of disgrace or shame associated with a particular characteristic of psychosis or psychotic condition. Stigma can lead to discrimination, prejudice, and social exclusion. Mental illness stigma is particularly pervasive and shameful and can have devastating consequences. The roots of stigma surrounding mental illness are deeply embedded in historical, cultural, and societal factors.

3. The source and origins of stigma

Stigma often originates from the way a society or community sees the condition or the disease, as regards whether it is normal (e.g., high blood pressure), contagious (e.g., some viral diseases), or abnormal (e.g., mental illnesses). The disapproval of the disease condition and the fear of harm predispose an individual to stigmatize an individual, to knowingly or unknowingly stigmatize a psychotic patient.

Historical and cultural factors that support or promote stigma:

1. History portrays mental illness as demonic possession or divine punishment. This is often rooted in beliefs in religious cycles and in communities. These beliefs determine the type of care or attention given to the patients with psychosis or living with psychosis. In most communities, patients with psychotic diseases are separated from society and may not receive medical or traditional attention. Some communities have cultural beliefs and/or practices that stigmatize mental illness, portraying mentally derailed persons as demonic and possessed individuals who are capable of attacking others with their spiritual powers. Media or community spokespersons may portray psychotic patients with comments that perpetuate negative stereotypes [3]. The cultural comparison on mental health perception and stigma in different communities varies, as shown in **Table 1**. This may vary across cultural groups, informed by cultures within a larger culture (Asians have many cultures embedded in their collective culture).

Cultural group	Perception of mental illness	Impact on stigma
Asian	Seen as a sign of personal weakness or failure of self-control	Stigma leads to family shame, discourages help-seeking
African	Attributed to spiritual or supernatural causes	High stigma levels, deter individuals from seeking psychiatric help
Arab	Viewed as a form of divine punishment	Significant stigma, leads to delayed or avoided treatment
Latin American	Attributed to personal weakness or lack of willpower	Stigmatizes individuals, discourages them from seeking psychiatric care
Western	Misconceptions about danger or unpredictability	Results in social exclusion and discrimination

Extracted from Ahad et al. [3].

Table 1.
A cultural comparison on mental health perception and stigma.

2. Lack of understanding and misinformation: The behaviors of patients with psychosis are often so strange to the people in the community/family that they ascribe it to spiritual beings. Their understanding of the cause of the disease condition is poor. This informs their reaction to patients with such conditions. There is limited public understanding of mental illness. This may be due to be unusual presentations, confessions, attacks/episodes, and so on. Presentations with element of aggression, vocalization of incomprehensible words, and abnormal posture are ascribed to deity role in a psychotic patient. In some communities, this earns psychotics undue popularity. The patients are seen as Godsend or as someone who possess divine powers. Patients are sometimes consulted for divination or insights into issues they feel are beyond human powers. Limited public understanding of mental illness can lead to misconceptions and negative attitudes. Some individuals may possess exceptional potentials that may be judged beneficial to communities (for example, the ability to say things that cannot be decoded, or ability see what others cannot see).

3. Misconceptions about the causes, symptoms, and treatment of psychosis: Most communities and religious circles uphold the belief that a human being is under the influence of spiritual beings. If the spiritual being is good or has good disposition, the person it inhabits will exhibit good characters and behaviors, but if the spirit is the bad or evil, the subject will exhibit bad behaviors and characters. The belief in the contagious nature of spirits reinforces the idea that these spirits can transfer from one person to another. This fear and misunderstanding often lead to avoidance and discrimination. Avoidance and discrimination are key elements of stigma, which make patients feel unwanted. Throughout history, mental illness has been misunderstood and often attributed to supernatural forces, demonic possession, or divine punishment. Cultural beliefs and practices shape attitudes toward mentally ill patients, leading to stigmatization and discrimination.

4. Media portrayals: Media often portrays individuals with mental illness in a negative or sensationalized manner, reinforcing stereotypes and fueling fear. Inaccurate or misleading portrayals of mental illness can contribute to stigma. This is often a result of misinformation or the illiteracy of the media personnel.

3.1 Types of stigma

Stigma is an act perpetrated by someone to harm another person; it may be intentional or unintentional. It can be from self, other persons, or a group of people.

1. Self-stigma: Some psychotic patients are aware of their actions and behaviors and can interpret such behaviors as abnormal. This often leads to self-stigma, evident in the patient's withdrawal from friends and society. Self-stigma results from the internalization of negative stereotypes by the patient and the patient's beliefs about himself. These negative beliefs cause low self-esteem and low self-efficacy and increase the feeling of shame and guilt. This can be traumatic and worsen the health status of the patient. The criticism by the public, blaming them for their inability to work [6] and integrate in the public, could result in self-stigma, which is evident in their withdrawal from social gatherings, work, or school.

2. Social stigma: It refers to the rejection of a psychotic patient by friends, associates, employers, and/or social media associates. It is about negative stereotypes, prejudice, and discrimination toward individuals or groups and, in this case, toward a mentally ill patient [7]. Social media bullying is common and can worsen the situation. Social stigma often leads to: discrimination and prejudice from others, limited social opportunities and support networks, and difficulty finding and maintaining employment and housing. The patient sees himself as an outcast. This uncertainty results in the fear of the unknown. Lack of understanding can lead to fear and avoidance of individuals with mental illness.

3. Healthcare stigma: Some healthcare workers sometimes put aside their training knowledge to believe that psychosis is contagious [8, 9]. There is also fear of harm by the patients. These fears contribute to unwillingness to attend to patients with psychosis. Most psychotic patents sense these actions and are reluctant to seek help due to fear of judgment and discrimination. They are unwilling to seek further medical attention because of the outcome of previous treatments and encounters, delayed treatment and poorer treatment outcomes, and stigmatizing attitudes among healthcare providers.

Stigma by healthcare professionals operates on three inter-related levels: a. structural, b. interpersonal, and c. intrapersonal [9]. Structural stigma refers to discriminatory healthcare structures, policy, and legislation [8, 9]. This is evident in health disparities for some populations (mentally ill persons) [10]. These disparities are seen in the budgetary allocation for mental health unit and the number of professionals specializing in mental health. Interpersonal stigma occurs as a result of negative interaction between health professionals in the mental health unit and other health professionals in the health institution. The interpersonal interaction with people with mental illness is shaped by cultural beliefs of the other health professionals they interact with. Negative beliefs negatively impact their interaction with mental health patients. This in turn affects the level of care given to these groups of patients. Interpersonal stigma is often caused by ignorance or misinformation, which affects the professionals' attitudes (prejudice) and behavior (targeted violence, discrimination, hostility, and human rights abuses) [11]. The attitude of mental healthcare professionals may be affected by the way the general public portray them and relate with them. For example, they may believe that people who relate with mad people are possessed by demons; this results in withdrawal of other health professionals from mental health professionals in public for fear of contamination by demons. These actions consciously or unconsciously affect the professionals. Intrapersonal stigma is revealed by the treatment by the patient of himself or other patients. Such behaviors have roots from their hospital experiences. Such stigma encompasses negative beliefs about themselves, which are largely based on shame, the acceptance of mental illness stereotypes, a sense of alienation from others, and consequent low mood. Positioning their ward far from other wards may also contribute to intrapersonal stigma.

3.2 Sources of stigma

Stigma can arise from various factors, including:

1. Lack of understanding and misinformation: People with limited knowledge of mental illnesses tend to judge based on their limited knowledge or instincts. Their little understanding of the nature of mental illness leads to misconceptions and fear. Inaccurate Information produces unacceptable actions. Misinformation about psychosis spreads through history, media, or personal experiences. This creates negative attitudes and stereotypes. Fear of the unknown or uncertainty often leads to misjudgment. Lack of understanding can lead to fear and avoidance of individuals with mental illness.

2. Historical and cultural factors: Historical stigma is often passed on from one generation to another. Historical portrayals of mental illness as demonic possession or divine punishment have left lasting negative impression on people/associations. Cultural beliefs and practices may stigmatize mental illness, leading to discrimination and social exclusion. There is a general thought that being mentally ill carries a connotation of shame and weakness of character [3, 5].

3. Media portrayals: Media often portrays individuals with mental illness in a negative or sensationalized manner, reinforcing stereotypes and fueling fear. Inaccurate or misleading portrayals of mental illness can contribute to stigma.

4. Social and economic factors: Discrimination based on mental illness can lead to social exclusion, limited opportunities, and difficulty accessing healthcare and employment. Individuals with mental illness may face economic hardship, which can further contribute to stigma.

5. Personal experiences: Negative personal experiences with individuals with mental illness can shape negative attitudes and beliefs. The fear that mental illness is contagious leads to avoidance and discrimination. A person who has been harmed by a mentally ill patient is likely to avoid them; this may be seen as stigmatization.

6. Self-stigma: Individuals with mental illness may internalize negative stereotypes and beliefs about themselves, leading to low self-esteem and self-doubt.

4. The role of stigma in exacerbating psychotic symptoms

Stigma exacerbates psychotic symptoms, thereby worsening the impact on society. Roles of stigma in psychosis include:

1. Stress and anxiety: The constant fear of stigma can lead to increased stress and anxiety. A psychotic patient is aware of his or her environment. Hostile environments make the patient anxious and ashamed of the condition. This makes him restless and stressed. Stress and anxiety exacerbate psychotic symptoms by making some of the brain centers unstable. Constant fear of stigma can cause retraction, which may aggravate depression and hinder socialization. The patient becomes locked in their thoughts and the thought of hatred by the people around them. Stress and anxiety exacerbate psychotic symptoms, complicate psychosis, and hinder recovery [12].

2. Social isolation: Most people do not want to associate with psychotic patients for fear of being hurt or because of the wrong notion that it is contagious (spirits can jump from one person to another). This singular action results in the isolation of a psychotic patient. Anytime the patient is welcomed, he is often bullied and made uncomfortable in their association. This attitude worsens psychotic symptoms and aggravates psychosis. Stigma can lead to social isolation, depriving individuals of support and understanding. These can contribute to feelings of loneliness and depression, which can worsen psychotic symptoms.

3. Non-adherence to treatment: Drugs used for the management of psychosis have noticeable, inconveniencing side effects. Such presentations cause stigma and fear of transmission to people close to the patients, resulting in people staying at a distance and avoiding the subject. To avoid this ugly situation, patients tend to avoid the medication to stay "normal" and accessible. Fear of stigma often leads to non-adherence to medication and therapy, resulting in poorer treatment outcomes and increased risk of relapse.

4.1 Effects of stigma on psychotic patients

There is a strong correlation between stigma, mental health, and negative outcomes.

Continual stigmatization of psychotic patients often leads to:

1. Increased risk of suicide: Stigma can lead to feelings of isolation, shame, and hopelessness, increasing the risk of suicide among individuals with mental illness.

2. Delayed treatment: Stigma can deter people from seeking help, leading to delayed or inadequate treatment, which can exacerbate mental health conditions and increase the risk of complications.

3. Poorer quality of life: Stigma can negatively impact social relationships, employment opportunities, and overall quality of life, contributing to poorer mental

health outcomes. As a result of stigma, people with mental illness are robbed of the opportunities that define a quality life: good jobs, safe housing, satisfactory healthcare, and affiliation with a diverse group of people [13].

5. Strategies to reduce stigma and improve outcomes

1. Education and awareness: Illiteracy is a disease, says an adage. Knowledge and understanding clears doubts and worries. Promoting public education about mental illness can dispel myths and misconceptions, challenge negative stereotypes, and foster empathy and understanding. Programs aimed at educating communities on psychosis and its presentation are important to reduce stigma and segregation. Proper awareness campaigns will erode traditional beliefs that psychosis is contagious. Educational campaigns can counter the pre-existing idea that mentally ill people are violent murderers by presenting statistics showing that homicide rates are similar among people with mental illness and the general public [14]. This will improve the public acceptance of people living with psychosis. Psychotic patients should be well tutored on the need to accept the condition as a kind of illness, not a spiritual spell. This alone will encourage patients to submit themselves for medical expert examination and treatment, thus resolving or improving their health statue. Frantic effort to promote public education about mental illness to dispel myths and misconceptions should be made continuously. Negative stereotypes must be challenged with the aim of promoting understanding and empathy. Steps to educate the public should include: Launching public health campaigns to raise awareness about mental health and challenge stigma, including mental health education in school curriculum, and the use of fliers to disseminate information on psychosis. Workplace training can be organized from time to time to raise workers' understating of psychosis and its presentations and possible side effects of medications used in its management. Provide mental health training to employers and employees to promote understanding and reduce workplace stigma. Public Service Announcements can effectively challenge stereotypes and promote understanding of mental illness. Announcements can be disseminated through various media channels, including television, radio, and social media. Anti-stigma training of healthcare providers to recognize and challenge stigma can help to create a more supportive and inclusive healthcare environment

2. Media advocacy: Promote media literacy to help people critically evaluate media portrayals of mental illness. Education and awareness of the media crews is important to change the type of programs they mount. Responsible media coverage of mental illness should be encouraged to help to reduce stigma and promote positive portrayals of individuals with mental illness. This will also positively affect the way they organize their programs and presentations. Responsible media coverage of mental illnesses must be encouraged. Deliberate efforts must be made to promote positive portrayals of individuals with mental illness and collaborate with media organizations to promote accurate and sensitive portrayals of mental illness. Patients who have returned from rehabilitation must be properly integrated into society. Non-governmental organizations and government agencies that support mental health advocacy to raise awareness and advocate for policy change should be encouraged.

3. Arts and culture: Mental health-themed art could raise public awareness. Using art, music, and literature to express mental health experiences can help to reduce stigma and promote empathy. Encouraging accurate and sensitive portrayals of mental illness in film and television can help to challenge stereotypes.

4. Social media campaigns: Social media can be used to raise awareness and challenge stigma. Social influencer collaboration to promote mental health awareness is a possible way of reducing stigma.

5. Policy and legislation: Laws that discourage stigma should be enacted, and proper legislation should be put in place. Institutions that are saddled with the responsibility of caring for the sick should advocate for policies that protect the rights of individuals with mental illness and support initiatives that promote mental health parity and reduce discrimination. Laws to be enacted could include: mental health parity laws—enact and enforce laws that require equal coverage for mental health and substance use disorder benefits—and anti-discrimination laws—strengthen anti-discrimination laws to protect individuals with mental illness from discrimination in employment, housing, and other areas [15]. Policy and system-level changes that impact positively mental health stigma should be encouraged, for example, health insurance reform: Continue advocating for policies that improve access to mental health care and reduce financial barriers. Criminal justice reform: Implement reforms to address the mental health needs of individuals involved in the criminal justice system and reduce the use of incarceration as a solution for mental health crises.

6. Community-based programs: Community-based programs that provide support, resources, and opportunities for social interaction can help to reduce stigma and improve the quality of life for individuals with psychosis. Efforts must be made to develop community-based programs that provide support and resources to individuals with psychosis. Programs that identify those with psychosis and provide a social link should be put in place. This will encourage sharing of ideas and experiences. Some community-based interventions include: peer support groups (to provide a safe and supportive environment for individuals with mental illness), community mental health centers (provide a range of services, including counseling, medication management, and case management), cultural competency training centers (produce culturally competent personnel to provide mental health services), personal stories and testimonials (encourage individuals with mental illness to share their stories and outcomes), celebrity advocacy (support celebrities and public figures to help raise awareness), and faith-based initiatives (collaborating with religious leaders to promote mental health awareness).

7. Workplace initiatives: Mental health training for employers and employees should be mounted on a regular basis. Workers are trained to recognize and respond to mental health issues in the workplace. This can help to create a more supportive environment. Programs that offers EAPs (Employee Assistance Programs) provide employees with access to mental health services and reduce stigma.

8. Global collaboration: International partnerships help to share ideas on the control of stigma. Collaboration with international organizations to share best

practices and coordinate efforts to reduce stigma can lead to more effective strategies, foster a global understanding of mental health issues, and create a unified approach to combating stigma worldwide. Global mental health initiatives help in decision making and management of psychotic patients. Keying into global initiatives that prioritize mental health and address stigma on a global scale and device is a way of addressing stigma.

9. Person-centered care: Care programs that are patient centered should be developed. This will erode the feeling of inadequate attention and the feeling of healthcare stigma among patients. The needs and preferences of individuals with psychosis should be prioritized. Psychotic patients should be given the opportunity to relate socially with healthcare providers. Prioritizing the needs and preferences of individuals with psychosis and fostering collaborative relationships between healthcare providers and patients can help to reduce stigma and improve treatment outcomes.

10. Innovative approaches: Technology-based interventions could reduce stigma. Utilizing technology, such as mobile apps and telehealth, could provide accessible mental health services and reduce stigma. Virtual reality therapy refocuses patient's attention. Exploring the use of virtual reality to expose individuals to virtual experiences that challenge stereotypes and promote empathy may be helpful in tackling stigma.

11. Research and innovation: Increase funding for mental health research to advance understanding of mental illness, develop effective treatments, and manage stigma. Develop and implement innovative interventions, such as technology-based interventions, to improve access to mental healthcare and reduce stigma.

12. Protest and advocacy

    Protest strategies are rooted in promoting civil rights agendas; protest strategies are formal objection to negative representations of people with mental illness or the nature of these illnesses. Grassroot-level protests by people who have experienced discrimination and/or by advocates on their behalf could be in the form of product rejection, letter writing, or public demonstrations [16]. The aim of protest is typically to remove negative representations or content or to suppress negative attitudes. The goal to enhance or enact protections of rights, increase access to social resources, and reduce inequalities is often the reason for protest that focuses on legislative reform. Protest often serves as a platform to increase public awareness and/or policy recognition of issues and concerns related to mental health [16].

5.1 Types of stigmas that reflect different survival concerns and methods of social surveillance

It is important to manage stigma as soon as it is diagnosed. The type of stigma often determines the management. Types of stigmas reflect different survival concerns for the reference group (the likelihood to commit suicide). This informs the management strategy and type of social surveillance. The different methods for the management of stigma require specific countertactics to address modes of operations of stigma and help proffer solution to stigma.

Stigma types particularly relevant for persons with mental illnesses include the following:

Apart from mental illness, people are stigmatized for other reasons of disease conditions. People living with communicable diseases, like AIDS and leprosy, are also stigmatized. There is need to ascertain the reason for the observed stigma. Some of the types of stigmas suffered by mental health patients include:

1. *Peril stigma*: Peril stigma is the stigma that triggers the urge to fight back. It is caused by the perception of potential danger. The stigmatized often shows odd, impulsive, or unpredictable behaviors, which may include attacks on people (those stigmatizing them or innocent people) or object (destruction of items around them to register their displeasure). These actions are sometimes prompted by defensive action to refrain from stigma or deter the people stigmatizing them.

2. *Moral stigma*: This is seen when the group that the patient associates with feels challenged (by exhibiting boldness more than them) by the patient. The mentally ill is perceived as a threat to the group for challenging the group's beliefs and values. Such stigma predisposes the patient to symptoms seen in some mental illnesses. The avoidance of the negative symptoms of psychosis, apathy of depression, or behavioral avoidance of anxiety disorders may trigger moral stigma, especially when interpreted as unwillingness to take responsibility or laziness, unwillingness to accept personal responsibility for one's life, or lack of predictable conformity to social rules of engagement, in which case the patient is judged unruly.

3. *Disruption stigma*: This occurs when a person's behaviors or symptoms of his mental illness are interpreted as interfering with functioning of the family or work group. Interaction with persons living with physical disabilities may invoke disruption stigma because of concerns that their presentations may threaten professional and social obligations. Tending to that person's needs may disrupt professional and social obligations. Within healthcare systems, clinicians engage in disruption stigma when psychiatric patients are not given equal diagnostic vigilance or when their budget is used by another arm of the hospital or when patients are "dumped" onto other services that are not psychiatry related.

4. *Empathy fatigue*: It represents a form of stigma when friends, family members, and co-workers feel too distressed to relate closely with the patient's suffering, that is, a feeling that it is "too much emotional work." They tend to avoid or keep social distance from the mentally ill. Mental illnesses are in most cases associated with feelings of severe depression, anxiety, and chronic pain. These presentations weary the caregiver and may evoke empathy fatigue, in which case caregivers or associates feel they are doing too much for the patient and as a result are distressed and incapacitated. This may lead to withdrawal of services rendered to the patient, resulting in infrequent visits to the patient and delayed feeding and attention.

5. *Courtesy stigma*: It is stigma by association that occurs when they feel that association or proximity to the mentally ill will earn them disrespect that may result in loss of social status in the group or community [17]. Family members or mental health professionals are vulnerable to courtesy stigma by virtue of association with persons with mental illness. The associates feel others are looking down on or mocking them as a result of their interaction with the sick.

The most difficult of all stigmatizing processes to counter is perhaps *internalized stigma*, that is, to be able to psychologically talk the patient out of internalized stigma. Internalized stigma results when stigma of whatever specific type becomes a lens for self-perception that is judgmental, contemptuous, and dismissive [18]. Patients feel disgust for their identity as psychiatrically ill. Compassion for self is difficult to muster. Loss of self-esteem, a sense of alienation, social withdrawal, and self-hatred are common occurrences in such patients.

5.2 Scientific basis of empathy stigma

Social relationships are determined by the brain. The process involves separation of associations and determination of the one that best suit the person, a process achieved through categorical social cognition. During this process, the socio-biological systems stream information about specific social world via the rostral anterior cingulate gyrus. At the rostra anterior cingulated gyrus, the information is compared to the existing model of expectable reality that has been constructed by the prefrontal cortex from memory retrieval [19]. Expectable realities are constructed during learning or interaction (for example, specific instructions on what is good and evil). Detection of stigma in the environment probably generates conflict between incoming socio-biological information and the specific expectable reality. Detection of such conflict by the anterior cingulate gyrus results in additional control signals to the prefrontal cortex. The incoming conflict detected by the dorsolateral and ventrolateral prefrontal cortices is processed by the same (by the dorsolateral and ventrolateral prefrontal cortices) to resolve the conflict by exercising top-down modulation over subcortical systems that constitute the pain matrix, including the amygdala (fear), insula (disgust), and ventral anterior cingulate gyrus (suffering) [19–21]. This leads to the activation of the pain matrix, which in turn produces proximate signals for avoiding or extruding the bearer of the stigmatizing mark. The signal information flow in the mirror neuron information is then suppressed. The suppression results in person-to-person social cognition failure or inactivation. Person-to-person social cognition failure results in the suspension of empathy for the stigmatized person. The stigmatized person is then behaviorally extruded and oppressed, for which the stigmatizer typically feels no guilt [22].

Different types of stigmas recruit different brain circuits and signaling pathways. Moral stigma, for examples, recruits circuitry of ventromedial prefrontal cortex that is essential for generating social disgust [23]. This is buttressed by loss of patient's aversion to intimate contact observed in patients with damage to the ventromedial prefrontal cortex. They find it difficult to relate with strangers, social deviants, or those bearing misfortunes, such as the poor or homeless, whereas their moral disgust remained intact for those who violated the dignity of others, with unfairness, cheating, or betrayal [23].

5.3 Management of stigma and interventions to counter stigma

Stigma is managed by initiating activities that can positively alter the categorical processes of person-to-person interaction, which is organized out of the mirror neuron system and medial prefrontal systems for mentalization and empathy. This system is "slow"; it permits a highly individualized appraisal of another person's actions/behaviors from a cognitive processing perspective and tunes individual emotions [24]. It is possible to reduce mirror neuron mediated empathy through physician training, and patients' experience sometimes reduces mirror neuron mediated empathy [25]. This evidence is supported by the finding that non-medical participants in training showed different patterns of event-related brain potentials (ERP) when witnessing people experiencing painful vs. non-painful stimuli, whereas internal medicine physicians showed no ERP differences when watching persons experiencing painful vs. non-painful stimuli. Reciprocal inhibition between person-to-person social cognition and categorical social cognition, which would potentially reestablish some aspects of empathy, provide a major strategy for countering interpersonal stigma. When a personal relationship is established with another person, categorical perception of that person predictably fades from attention, because he tends to trust the person with whom he has established relationship. These pathways may likely explain the effectiveness of social contact/exposure in anti-stigma interventions that facilitate interaction between potential stigmatizers and persons with mental illness in recovery and explain the importance of psychotherapy [14]. Establishing person-to-person positive interactions with a potential stigmatizer as quickly as possible is thus a high priority for a person at risk of stigmatization. The processes should include the training or enlightenment of the stigmatizer on the mental health challenges. The earlier the better.

A second strategy is embedded in the relationship between high arousal states and a bias toward categorical social cognition. Activation of the anterior cingulate gyrus by perception of a stigmatizing mark activates not only the prefrontal cortex but also the ventrolateral tegmentum (dopaminergic pathways) and locus coeruleus (noradrenergic pathways). These monoamine systems ascend to cortical and limbic regions where their modulation heightens brain arousal, primes the orienting reflex, and re-allocates attention for sensitized detection of marks of stigma [19]. Arousal due to ambiguity, threat, or uncertainty will produce a shift toward categorical social cognition. Conversely, a lowering of arousal produces a shift toward person-to-person social cognition. Lowering arousal is achieved by reducing ambiguity, reducing perception of threat, and bolstering a sense of coherence and predictability about the potential stigmatizer's circumstances.

Psychiatrists must activate person-to-person social cognition and diminish alertness to threat. These will together form the bedrock for building strategies to counter stigma in interpersonal interactions [26].

6. Counseling as a tool for resolving stigma

Counseling can be a powerful tool in addressing and resolving stigma, particularly in the context of mental health. This can be achieved by:

1. Understanding and challenging stigma: Understanding the type of stigma a patient is facing is crucial to resolving stigma-related issues. Subjects must have a clear picture of the kind/type of sickness from which they are suffering. Counselors provide accurate information about mental health conditions, debunking myths and misconceptions. Counselors, through interaction with the patient, identify their concerns and challenges and counsel the patient on the challenges identified. These challenges and concerns could be a significant barrier to seeking help, which in turn could affect recovery. Addressing patients' personal biases helps resolve psychiatric illnesses. Taking patients through empathy-building exercises can remove the patient's thoughts/mind from the source of concerns

and self-stigma. Counselors can help clients develop a deeper understanding of the experiences of others, reducing prejudice and discrimination.

2. Building self-esteem and self-efficacy through counseling: This helps to resolve psychotic issues by removing related stigma and improve patient's medical attention-seeking and compliance to prescribed treatment protocols. Psychotherapy has been known to be a useful tool for resolving some form of psychosis. These can be achieved through counseling by:

   a. Enhance self-worth: Counselors can help clients build self-esteem by emphasizing their strengths and accomplishments.

   b. Promote self-efficacy: Setting achievable goals and celebrating successes are one of several tools used by counselors to empower clients to believe in their ability to overcome challenges.

   c. Challenging negative self-talk: Counselors can help clients identify and replace negative thoughts with positive thoughts and affirmations.

3. Developing coping strategies: Counselors are exposed to techniques of developing coping strategies. Some techniques are:

   a. Stress management techniques: Counselors teach clients effective stress management techniques, such as mindfulness, meditation, and deep breathing.

   b. Social skills training: By improving social skills counselors can help clients build stronger relationships and reduce social isolation.

   c. Problem-solving skills: Counselors can teach clients problem-solving skills to help them navigate challenges and overcome obstacles.

4. Advocacy and empowerment: Useful interaction with a patient often unfolds the cause of the illness, especially if it is a result of stress induced by lacks (of job, money, relationships). Patient can be helped by:

   a. Encouraging help-seeking: Counselors can encourage clients to seek help from mental health professionals and other support services.

   b. Advocacy training: Counselors can empower clients to advocate for their own needs and challenge stigma within their communities.

   c. Community engagement: Counselors can facilitate community-based initiatives to raise awareness about mental health and reduce stigma.

7. Cultural considerations in counseling for stigma

Cultural factors significantly influence how individuals perceive and respond to mental health issues. Counselors must be attuned to these cultural nuances to effectively address stigma and provide culturally competent care.

1. Some key considerations are:

    a. Cultural beliefs and values: Cultural stigma varies widely from one culture to another. The gravity of cultural stigma depends on how strong the belief is. Some cultures may view mental illness as spiritual or physical weakness; others may normalize it as a natural part of life, while others may idolize it and sense it as beneficial to society.

    b. Help-seeking behaviors: Cultural norms can influence help-seeking behaviors. Some cultures may encourage seeking help from family, religious leaders, or traditional healers, while others may prioritize individual coping mechanisms. The advent of orthodox medicine has strongly impacted these beliefs.

    c. Communication styles: Different cultures have varying communication styles, including directness, indirectness, and emotional expression. Understanding these differences is crucial for effective therapeutic communication.

2. Cultural sensitivity and humility: Counselors should be conversant with the cultural beliefs in the community and should not be influenced by such cultural beliefs, and counselors should strive to develop cultural competence, which involves understanding and respecting diverse cultural backgrounds. Counselors should be aware of their own cultural biases and assumptions.

3. Culturally appropriate interventions. Cultural interventions must be complete and encompassing. The involvement of family and traditional healer sometimes boasts the confidence of the patient and improves outcomes. The opinion of the patient must be sought before inclusion of a family member in their care system. Communication skill is also very important in counseling. Communicating in the language that the patient is comfortable with improves outcomes.

8. Evidence-based interventions for stigma reduction

Evidence-based interventions have been developed to address stigma and promote mental health. These interventions target various levels, including individual, community, and societal. Effective approaches include:

1. Individual-level interventions

    a. Cognitive behavioral therapy (CBT): CBT can help individuals challenge negative thoughts and beliefs about mental illness, reducing self-stigma and improving self-esteem.

    b. Motivational interviewing: This technique can help individuals increase motivation to seek help and engage in treatment, reducing barriers related to stigma.

    c. Psychosocial interventions: These interventions can help individuals develop coping skills, social skills, and problem-solving abilities, enhancing their resilience and reducing the impact of stigma.

2. Community-level interventions

   a. Stigma reduction campaigns: Public awareness campaigns can challenge stereotypes, promote understanding, and reduce stigma.

   b. Community education and training: Educating community members, including healthcare providers, teachers, and law enforcement, can increase knowledge and reduce stigma.

   c. Peer support groups: Peer support groups provide a safe and supportive environment for individuals with mental illness to share experiences, reduce isolation, and challenge stigma.

3. Societal-level interventions

   a. Anti-discrimination legislation: Laws and policies that protect the rights of individuals with mental illness can help to reduce stigma and discrimination.

   b. Media advocacy: Promoting accurate and positive media portrayals of mental illness can challenge stereotypes and reduce stigma.

   c. Policy advocacy: Advocating for policies that support mental health services and research can help to reduce stigma and improve access to care.

8.1 Medications for resolving stigma

Medication itself does not directly resolve stigma. These medications indirectly contribute to reducing stigma by:

a. Improving functioning: Effective medication can help individuals manage symptoms, improve their quality of life, and function better in society. This can challenge negative stereotypes and misconceptions about mental illness.

b. Reducing the burden of symptoms: By alleviating symptoms like depression, anxiety, or psychosis, medication can help individuals participate more fully in social and work activities, reducing stigma associated with these conditions or inability to perform or participate.

c. Normalizing treatment: Openly discussing the use of medication for mental health conditions can help to normalize treatment and reduce the stigma associated with seeking help. For example, discussing the possible side effects of the drugs and reassuring the patients that it will wear away as soon as the patient improves and the dose is reduced.

9. Challenges in stigma reduction

While significant progress has been made in reducing stigma associated with mental illness, numerous challenges persist:

1. Lack of awareness and understanding:

    a. Misconceptions and myths: Persistent misconceptions and myths about mental illness continue to fuel stigma.

    b. Limited mental health literacy: Many people lack basic knowledge about mental health conditions, leading to misunderstanding and fear.

2. Social stigma and discrimination:

    a. Social exclusion: Individuals with mental illness often face social exclusion and discrimination, leading to isolation and reduced quality of life.

    b. Workplace discrimination: Stigma can hinder employment opportunities and career advancement.

3. Healthcare system barriers:

    a. Limited access to care: Inadequate access to mental health services, particularly in underserved areas, can exacerbate stigma.

    b. Discriminatory practices: Discriminatory attitudes and practices within healthcare settings can discourage individuals from seeking help.

4. Cultural and religious barriers:

    a. Cultural stigma: Cultural beliefs and practices can perpetuate stigma, especially in cultures that view mental illness as a sign of weakness or shame.

    b. Religious stigma: Religious beliefs may contribute to stigma by associating mental illness with sin or demonic possession.

5. Media portrayals:

    a. Negative stereotypes: Media often portrays individuals with mental illness in a negative or sensationalized manner, reinforcing stereotypes.

    b. Sensationalized coverage: Sensationalized coverage of violence or crime committed by individuals with mental illness can further stigmatize the entire group.

10. Advances in stigma reduction

While the challenges associated with mental health stigma are significant, there are also numerous opportunities to reduce stigma and promote mental health. One of the key advancements in the control and management of stigma-induced health challenges are the use of products of technological advancement.

10.1 Technological advancements in the management of stigma

a. Telehealth: The rise of telehealth has made mental health services more accessible, reducing barriers to care and potentially reducing stigma [27].

b. Mobile apps: Mental health apps can provide support, education, and self-help tools, empowering individuals and reducing stigma.

c. Online platforms are being developed to provide mental health support, education, and community.

d. Virtual reality therapy: Virtual reality experiences can be used to challenge stereotypes and promote empathy [28].

e. Mindfulness and meditation apps: These apps offer tools to manage stress, anxiety, and depression, reducing stigma associated with seeking help [29, 30].

f. Neurobiological research: Ongoing research is advancing our understanding of the biological basis of mental illness, leading to more effective treatments and reducing stigma.

g. Personalized medicine: Tailored treatments based on individual genetic and biological factors can improve outcomes and reduce the negative impact of mental illness.

h. Neurofeedback: Training individuals to regulate their brainwave patterns can improve attention, focus, and mood [31].

i. Transcranial magnetic stimulation (TMS): Using TMS can help target specific brain regions involved in mood regulation, anxiety, and depression [32].

j. Deep brain stimulation (DBS): Implanting electrodes in the brain can help stimulate specific areas, often used for severe treatment-resistant depression and obsessive-compulsive disorder [33].

10.2 Support for stigmatized psychotic patients

A number of resources are available for stigmatized psychotic patients. These resources could assist in resolving stigma in mentally ill patients. The resources available are for the mentally ill patient and their caregiver. Some of these resources are:

- World Health Organization (WHO): The WHO has a wealth of information on mental health and stigma. This information could help inform the ill and their caregiver and the community as well.

- National Alliance on Mental Illness (NAMI): NAMI provides resources and support for individuals with mental illness and their families.

- Mental Health America (MHA): MHA works to promote mental health and reduce stigma.

It is important to remember that mental illness is a treatable condition, and with the right support, individuals can recover and live a fulfilling live. They can blend well with society and function optimally to the benefit of society. There are books that address stigma and its reduction strategies. Such books are available in hard and soft copies. Link to such resources will impact positively on the patient, their families, and the entire community.

The World Health Organization (WHO) has extensively addressed the issue of stigma related to mental health. They have published various reports and guidelines highlighting the detrimental effects of stigma and advocating for strategies to reduce stigma.

Here are some key WHO initiatives and reports related to stigma:

- The Overwhelming Case for Ending Stigma and Discrimination in Mental Health: This 2022 report, produced by the Lancet Commission, provides a comprehensive overview of the evidence on stigma and discrimination in mental health. It outlines the harmful effects of stigma and offers recommendations for reducing it [34, 35].

- Quality Rights Initiative: This initiative aims to improve the quality of mental healthcare and promote human rights. It includes strategies to combat stigma and discrimination, such as training healthcare providers and raising public awareness [36].

- Mental Health Action Plan 2013–2030: This global plan outlines strategies to improve mental health worldwide, including addressing stigma and discrimination [37].

Currently, WHO has taken some steps to reduce stigma. Some of their steps are:

The Lancet Commission provides eight recommendations for various stakeholders, including WHO, on what to do to reduce stigma and discrimination. Both Graham and Charlene have been working to implement these recommendations [35].

Global Mental Health Peer Network, an organization that was founded by Charlene, has taken ownership of recommendation 8—developing funded programs for people with lived experience [35]. The Global Mental Health Peer Network has empowered people living with mental health conditions to break down stigma in their communities and countries by providing them with a peer community and training opportunities [35, 38]. The inclusion of people with mental health conditions in the fight against stigma (in employment, education, communities) will go a long way to tell the story. By including people with stigma, deserving of dignity and human rights, which others see as another human being, will go a long way to reduce stigma.

Graham and other researchers in King's College London have partnered with WHO/Europe and members of the Global Mental Health Peer Network to fulfill recommendation 2, by developing a toolkit to reduce stigma and discrimination in mental health.

The toolkit, which was launched in 2024, called the "WHO MOSAIC toolkit to end stigma and discrimination in mental health," which provides practical, step-by-step guidance on how to set up anti-stigma initiatives based on principles of social contact, co-leadership by people with lived experience, and meaningful collaboration. It aims to be useful for individuals as well as groups and organizations [39].

Author details

Sunday Oritsetimenyin Otimenyin[1*] and Esther Badugu Patrick[2]

1 Department of Pharmacology, Faculty of Pharmaceutical Sciences, University of Jos, Jos, Plateau State, Nigeria

2 Department of Pharmacology, Faculty of Pharmaceutical Sciences, Kaduna State, Kaduna, Nigeria

*Address all correspondence to: sundayotimenyin@gmail.com

References

[1] Henderson C et al. Mental health-related stigma in health care and mental health-care settings. The Lancet Psychiatry. 2014;**1**(6):467-482

[2] Arboleya-Faedo T et al. Experiences of self-stigma in people with chronic psychosis: A qualitative study. International Journal of Environmental Research and Public Health. 2023;**20**(9):5688

[3] Ahad AA et al. Understanding and addressing mental health stigma across cultures for improving psychiatric care: A narrative review. Cureus. 2023;**15**(5):e39549

[4] Radua J et al. What causes psychosis? An umbrella review of risk and protective factors. World Psychiatry. 2018;**17**(1):49-66. DOI: 10.1002/wps.20490

[5] Arboleda-Flórez J. What causes stigma? World Psychiatry. 2002;**1**(1):25-26

[6] Stuart H, Arboleda-Florez J. Community attitudes toward people with schizophrenia. Canadian Journal of Psychiatry. 2001;**46**:245-452

[7] Luo H, Li Y, Yang BX, Chen J, Zhao P. Psychological interventions for personal stigma of patients with schizophrenia: A systematic review and network meta-analysis. Journal of Psychiatric Research. 2022;**148**:348-356. DOI: 10.1016/j.jpsychires.2022.02.010. Epub 2022 Feb 16

[8] Schulze B, Angermeyer MC. Subjective experiences of stigma. A focus group study of schizophrenic patients, their relatives and mental health professionals. Social Science & Medicine. 2003;**56**:299-312

[9] Cook JE, Purdie-Vaughns V, Meyer IH, Busch JTA. Intervening within and across levels: A multilevel approach to stigma and public health. Social Science & Medicine. 2014;**103**:101-109

[10] Band-Winterstein T. Health care provision for older persons: The interplay between ageism and elder neglect. Journal of Applied Gerontology. 2013;**34**(3):NP113-NP127. DOI: 10.1177/0733464812475308

[11] Thornicroft G. Shunned: Discrimination against People with Mental Illness. Oxford: Oxford University Press; 2006. p. 32

[12] Moriarty A, Jolley S, Callanan M, Garety P. Understanding reduced activity in psychosis: The roles of stigma and views of illness psychosis. Social Psychiatry and Psychiatric Epidemiology. 2012;**47**:1685-1693

[13] Corrigan PW, Watson AC. (2002). Understanding the impact of stigma on people with mental illness. World Psychiatry. 2002;**1**(1):16-20

[14] Corrigan PW, Morris SB, Michaels PJ, Rafacz JD, Rüsch N. Challenging the public stigma of mental illness: A meta-analysis of outcome studies. Psychiatric Services. 2012;**63**(10):963-973. DOI: 10.1176/appi.ps.201100529

[15] Committee on the Science of Changing Behavioral Health Social Norms, Board on Behavioral, Cognitive, and Sensory Sciences, Division of Behavioral and Social Sciences and Education, National Academies of Sciences, Engineering, and Medicine. Ending Discrimination Against People with Mental and Substance Use Disorders: The Evidence for Stigma Change. Washington, DC: National Academies Press (US); 2016

[16] Arboleda-Flórez J, Stuart H. From sin to science: Fighting the stigmatization of mental illnesses. Canadian Journal of Psychiatry. 2012;**57**(8):457-463. DOI: 10.1177/070674371205700803

[17] Goffman E. Stigma: Notes on the Management of Spoiled Identity. Englewood Cliffs: Prentice-Hall; 1963

[18] Stuart H, Arboleda-Florez J, Sartorius N. Paradigms Lost: Fighting Stigma and the Lessons Learned. New York: Oxford University Press; 2012

[19] Botvinick M, Braver T, Barch D, et al. Conflict monitoring and cognitive control. Psychological Review. 2001;**108**:624-652. DOI: 10.1037/0033-295x.108.3.624

[20] Chiao JY. Neural basis of social status hierarchy across species. Current Opinion in Neurobiology. 2010;**20**:803-809. DOI: 10.1016/j.conb.2010.08.006

[21] Greene JD, Nystrom LE, Engell AD, et al. The neural bases of cognitive conflict and control in moral judgement. Neuron. 2004;**44**:389-400. DOI: 10.1016/j.neuron.2004.09.027

[22] Griffith JL. Religion that Heals, Religion That Harms: A Guide for Clinical Practice. New York: Guilford Press; 2010. pp. 36-55

[23] Chiaramelli E, Sperotto R, Mattioli F, et al. Damage to the ventromedial prefrontal cortext reduces interpersonal disgust. Social Cognitive and Affective Neuroscience. 2013;**8**:171-180. DOI: 10.1093/scan/nss087

[24] Griffith JL. Religion that Heals, Religion That Harms: A Guide for Clinical Practice. New York: Guilford Press; 2010. p. 1355

[25] Decety J, Yang C-Y, Cheng Y. Physicians down-regulate their pain empathy response: An event-related brain potential study. NeuroImage. 2010;**50**:1676-1682. DOI: 10.1016/j.neuroimage.2010.01.025

[26] Griffith JL, Kohrt BA. Managing stigma effectively: What social psychology and social neuroscience can teach us. Academic Psychiatry. 2016;**40**(2):339-347. DOI: 10.1007/s40596-015-0391-0. Epub 2015 Jul 11

[27] Couch JV, Whitcomb M, Buchheit BM, Dorr DA, Malinoski DJ, Korthuis PT, et al. Patient perceptions of and experiences with stigma using telehealth for opioid use disorder treatment: A qualitative analysis. Harm Reduction Journal. 2024;**21**(1):125. DOI: 10.1186/s12954-024-01043-5

[28] Yuen ASY, Mak WWS. The effects of immersive virtual reality in reducing public stigma of mental illness in the university population of Hong Kong: Randomized controlled trial. Journal of Medical Internet Research. 2021;**23**(7):e23683. DOI: 10.2196/23683

[29] Jacobsen P, Choksi T, Sawyer K, Maximen C, Harding E, Richardson M. Home practice in mindfulness-based interventions for psychosis groups: A systematic review and qualitative study. BMC Psychology. 2022;**10**(1):9. DOI: 10.1186/s40359-021-00694-4

[30] Macrynikola N, Mir Z, Gopal T, Rodriguez E, Li S, Cox M, et al. The impact of mindfulness apps on psychological processes of change: A systematic review. npj Mental Health Research. 2024;**3**(1):14. DOI: 10.1038/s44184-023-00048-5

[31] Patil AU, Lin C, Lee SH, Huang HW, Wu SC, Madathil D, et al. Review of EEG-based neurofeedback as a therapeutic intervention to treat

depression. Psychiatry Research: Neuroimaging. 2023;**329**:111591. DOI: 10.1016/j.pscychresns.2023.111591. Epub 2023 Jan 13

[32] Chen L, Klooster DCW, Tik M, Thomas EHX, Downar J, Fitzgerald PB, et al. Accelerated repetitive transcranial magnetic stimulation to treat major depression: The past, present, and future. Harvard Review of Psychiatry. 2023;**31**(3):142-161. DOI: 10.1097/HRP.0000000000000364

[33] Dandekar MP, Diaz AP, Rahman Z, Silva RH, Nahas Z, Aaronson S, et al. A narrative review on invasive brain stimulation for treatment-resistant depression. Brazilian Journal of Psychiatry. 2022;**44**(3):317-330. DOI: 10.1590/1516-4446-2021-1874

[34] World Health Organization. The Overwhelming Case for Ending Stigma and Discrimination in Mental Health. 26 Jun 2024. Available from: https://www.who.int/europe/news-room/26-06-2024-the-overwhelming-case-for-ending-stigma-and-discrimination-in-mental-health

[35] Thornicroft G, Sunkel C, Aliev AA, Baker S, Brohan E, El Chammay R, et al. The Lancet Commission on ending stigma and discrimination in mental health. Lancet. 2022;**400**(10361):1438-1480

[36] Funk M, Bold ND. WHO's quality rights initiative: Transforming services and promoting rights in mental health. Health and Human Rights. 2020;**22**(1):69-75

[37] World Health Organization. Comprehensive Mental Health Action Plan 2013-2030. 2021. Available from: https://iris.who.int/bitstream/handle/10665/345301/9789240031029-eng.pdf

[38] Sunkel C. The global mental health peer network. In: Okpaku SO, editor. Innovations in Global Mental Health. Cham: Springer; 2021. DOI: 10.1007/978-3-030-57296-9_96

[39] World Health Organization. Mosaic Toolkit to End Stigma and Discrimination in Mental Health. 2024. Available from: https://iris.who.int/bitstream/handle/10665/379124/9789289061384-eng.pdf?